PURE YOGA

Inge Engelmann
2016

Pure Yoga

A translation from the Sanskrit into English of the tāntric work, The Gheraṇḍasaṃhitā, with a guiding commentary by

YOGĪ PRAṆAVĀNANDA

Edited with Introduction by
TONY RODRIGUEZ
DR. KANSHI RAM

MOTILAL BANARSIDASS PUBLISHERS
PRIVATE LIMITED • DELHI

4th Reprint: Delhi, ***2016***
First Edition: Delhi, 1992

ISBN: 978-81-208-0922-2 (Cloth)
ISBN : 978-81-208-1508-7 (Paper)

Also available at:
MOTILAL BANARSIDASS
41 U.A. Bungalow Road, Jawahar Nagar, Delhi 110 007
8 Mahalaxmi Chamber, 22 Bhulabhai Desai Road, Mumbai 400 026
203 Royapettah High Road, Mylapore, Chennai 600 004
236, 9th Main III Block, Jayanagar, Bengaluru 560 011
8 Camac Street, Kolkata 700 017
Ashok Rajpath, Patna 800 004
Chowk, Varanasi 221 001

Printed in India
by RP Jain at NAB Printing Unit,
A-44, Naraina Industrial Area, Phase I, New Delhi–110028
and published by JP Jain for Motilal Banarsidass Publishers (P) Ltd,
41 U.A. Bungalow Road, Jawahar Nagar, Delhi-110007

DEDICATION

"To all Masters of Yoga, past, present and future, and, in a special way, to Śakti, my eternal companion, this work is truthfully dedicated, in loving reverence."

INVOCATION

O Living Flame of Love,
O Life Sublime,
Transcendent in your Immanent Splendour,
Abide, Abide with me!
Bring Forth the Eternal Harmony
In Waves of Blissful Joy—
The Light Communing with the Light Divine,
Searching the Depths of being,
Reverberating, Unalloyed,
Regenerated, Holy, Whole, Supreme.
Shine Forth! Shine Forth!
O Living Flame of Love,
O Life Sublime,
O Light Divine.
Shine Forth!. . .

"As fire which is one, entering this world becomes varied in shape according to the object (it burns), so also the one Self within all beings becomes varied according to whatever (it enters) and also exists outside (them all)."

(Kaṭha Upaniṣad II, ii, 9)

PREFACE

So many books on Yoga have appeared during the past fifty years or so, that the reader may well ask himself the question: Is there any need for yet another book on the subject? This is the sort of question which the present book attempts to answer. It seems to be in the very nature of Yoga to become different things to different people, with the result that, quite often, what used to be in the past a Sacred and Pure Science has simply become a very shallow and, sometimes, even a very unsightly thing; so far remote, in fact, from Yoga that it is virtually unrecognizable.

It has been said that "those people who do not know the real nature of human life, and as a result constantly pursue the objects of worldly desire, remain involved in the darkness of ignorance concerning the realities of life. In still greater darkness remain those who, mistaking theoretical knowledge concerning Reality for the Reality itself, are intent upon the pursuit of such knowledge without making earnest effort to find that Reality by direct Realization."[1]

How many times is Yoga pursued, by disciple and guru alike, simply as another form of worldly desire? How many times is it the object of a purely mental exercise and speculation? These two are the Scylla and Charybdis placed on opposite sides of the narrow straits of Yoga; it is very hard to steer clear of one without being caught by the other. More often than not, the voyager perishes at the fauces of the six-headed monster of world illusion, or disappears in the whirlpool of self-delusion.

The path of True Yoga leads out of the darkness into the light. It takes us up, where we now stand, and leads us unerringly unto heights of unimaginable splendour, where Love, Peace and Wisdom reign supreme. But the goal of Yoga can only be reached through a regenerated, spiritual mind; a mind which is pure and extremely sensitive to Life's highest purpose. It is written in Yoga-vāsiṣṭha: "There are two paths to destroy the fluctuations of the mind, namely Yoga and Jñāna (Wisdom). Yoga is that which makes the actions of the mind integrated. But Jñāna is that which enables one to enjoy happiness in all objects."[2]

Needless to say, the realized individual sees no real difference between these two, for Yoga is the heart of Jñāna, and this, in turn, the heart of Yoga.

The Gheraṇḍa-saṃhitā is a text on Yoga. It is not just a treatise on Haṭha-yoga, as most people have come to understand the meaning of the word 'haṭha' and as the reader will discover. It is Integral Yoga at its best. Some western traditions and commentators have, from time to time, referred to teachings like the one presented here, as 'decadent Indian and Tibetan methods'; some people, on the other hand, have taken themselves to the teachings and self-appointed gurus with such superficial naivety and unwise enthusiasm—even if sometimes sincere—that they almost automatically place themselves in no position to derive any real benefits from them, for they lack the key to the proper understanding of the Sacred Science. Every single time that Yoga is misunderstood, misconceived, it degenerates into something which is only Yoga by name, i.e. gymnastics, fakirism, beauty culture and therapy, health science, sex therapy, meditation technique and so on. Thus distorting it and even bringing the Sacred Science into disrepute. The problem is nothing new for, True Yoga, in ancient times "... was taught from father to son in the line of Kings who were Saints; but in the revolutions of times immemorial this doctrine was forgotten by men. Today I am revealing to thee this Yoga Eternal, this Secret Supreme, because of thy love for me, and because I am thy friend."[3] So spoke Kṛṣṇa to his beloved disciple many centuries ago. Though Eternal, Yoga is constantly being lost; it is also constantly being found. Wise indeed is he who finds it.

He whose approach to Yoga is pure, practical and consistent, will come to know Yoga. To him only the Secret Supreme can be revealed. Hence the title for this new translation of a most competent treatise—seldom properly understood—on the integral Science of Yoga: Pure Yoga. He who would aspire to reach the sublime heights of Rāja-yoga must, above all else, be pure.

A treatise such as the Gheraṇḍa-saṃhitā would be thoroughly misleading and virtually unintelligible without a guiding commentary. In preparing such a commentary the writer has drawn both upon his own experience and various reliable sources; normally, the older the source—allowing for the odd worthy exception—the more reliable. There is no claim here to any final authority. The only reliable proof of True Yoga is in Yoga; the purer the better.

The reader will find it useful and perhaps even illuminating to consult the various tables as he or she reads through the text.

YOGĪ PRAṆAVĀNANDA

THE SANSKRIT ALPHABET AND PRONUNCIATION

(Transliteration)

The order of the Sanskrit alphabet is as follows:

a, ā, i, ī, u, ū, ṛ, ṝ ḷ, e, ai, o, au, ṃ, ḥ, k, kh, g, gh, ṅ,
अ आ इ ई उ ऊ ऋ ॠ ऌ ए ऐ ओ औ ं ः क ख ग घ ङ

c, ch, j, jh, ñ, ṭ, ṭh, ḍ, ḍh, ṇ, t, th, d, dh, n, p, ph, b, bh,
च छ ज झ ञ ट ठ ड ढ ण त थ द ध न प फ ब भ

m, y, r, l, v, ś, ṣ, s, h
म य र ल व श ष स ह

Vowels

a, ā, i, ī, u, ū, ṛ, ṝ, ḷ, e, ai, o, au
अ आ इ ई उ ऊ ऋ ॠ ऌ ए ऐ ओ औ

ṃ (anusvāra) ं   ḥ (visarga) ः

Consonants

Gutturals or Velars:	ka क	kha ख	ga ग	gha घ	ṅa ङ
Palatals:	ca च	cha छ	ja ज	jha झ	ña ञ
Cerebral or Retroflex:	ṭa ट	ṭha ठ	ḍa ड	ḍha ढ	ṇa ण
Dentals:	ta त	tha थ	da द	dha ध	na न
Labials:	pa प	pha फ	ba ब	bha भ	ma म
Semivowels:	ya य	ra र	la ल	va व	
Sibilants:	śa श	ṣa ष	sa स		
Aspirate:	ha ह	’ (the apostrophe) ऽ			

Vowels *English equivalent*

a—like the a in organ or the u in but.

ā—like the a in far or father but held twice as long as short a.

i—like the i in pin or fit.

ī—like the i in pique or fee but held twice as long as short i.

u—like the u in push or put.

ū—like the u in rule but held twice as long as short u.

ṛ—like the ri in rim.

ṝ—like the ree in reed.

ḷ—like the l followed by ṛ (lṛ).

e—like the e in they.

ai—like the ai in aisle.

o—like the o in go or rope.

au—like the ow in how or found.

ṃ—a resonant nasal like the n in the French word bon.

ḥ—a final h-sound: aḥ is pronounced like aha; iḥ like ihi.

Consonants

k—as in kite or kill.

kh—as in Eckhart.

g—as in give.

gh—as in dig-holes.

ṅ—as in cling.

c—as in chair or chill.

ch—as in punch hard.

j—as in joy.

jh—as in hedgehog.

ñ—as in canyon.

ṭ—as in tub or try.
ṭh—as in right hand.
ḍ—as in dove.
ḍh—as in red-hot.
ṇ—as rna (prepare to say the r but say na)
} but with tongue to roof of mouth.

t—as in tub or try.
th—as in right hand.
d—as in dove.
dh—as in red-hot.
} but with tongue against the teeth.

n—as in nut but with tongue between the teeth.

p—as in pine or pill.

ph—as in uphill.

Consonants *English equivalent*

b—as in bond.
bh—as in sub-head.
m—as in mother.
y—as in yes.
r—as in ram.
l—as in light.
v—as in vine.
ś—as the sh in shine.
ṣ—as the s in the German word 'sprechen'.
s—as in son.
h—as in home.

Sanskrit syllables carry no strong accentuation, only a flowing of short and long (twice as long as the short) syllables.

CONTENTS

THE SECOND LESSON

THE THIRD LESSON

INTRODUCTION

THERE ARE SIX DARŚANAS, methods or perspectives in Hindu philosophy. They are known as: (1) Sāṃkhya, the cosmological or evolutionary approach which has as its method intellectual knowledge with emphasis on the classification of principles; (2) Vaiśeṣika, the naturalistic or experimental point of view, based on sensorial experience, propounder of the atomistic theory; (3) Nyāya, or the point of view of Logic, which has as its tool dialectics; (4) Yoga, with elaborate disciplines on the control and transcendence of the mind, senses and inner faculties; it relates to the unfoldment of intuition, the experience of mystical states and Self-realization; (5) Mīmāṃsā, or the ritualistic approach, with elaborate religious practices and strict adherence to the letter of revealed Scripture; the province of Karmakāṇḍa; and (6) Vedānta (in its three approaches, i.e. Dvaita, Viśiṣṭādvaita and Advaita) or the end of Wisdom, expounding the ultimate purpose of all Revelation, the end of the Vedas, the path of Jñāna, with rigorous emphasis on metaphysical enquiry. Of these six, Vedānta and Yoga are considered to be the two highest systems, the former depicting the essence of Truth and knowing; the latter, blazing a trail to direct personal experience of the truths of the former. So, it has been rightly said in the Yoga-śikhā Upaniṣad:

ज्ञानं केचिद्वदन्त्यत्र केवलं तन्न सिद्धये
योगहीनं कथं ज्ञानं मोक्षदं भवतीह भोः ।
ज्ञाननिष्ठो विरक्तोऽपि धर्मज्ञो विजितेन्द्रियः
विना योगेन देवोऽपि न मोक्षं लभते विधे ॥

"Some say that Jñāna is enough to attain salvation. O God Brahman, that of itself is not enough. How can that Jñāna devoid of Yoga conduce to salvation?
One would not, O Brahman, attain salvation without Yoga even though one be steadfast in Jñāna or thoroughly non-attached, or virtuous, or self-conquered, even if one be a god."

And the Yogabīja Upaniṣad also is totally unambiguous about the paramount importance of Yoga and the place it occupies in Hindu philosophy, as indicated by the following:

> प्रविचार्य चिरं ज्ञानान्मुक्तोऽहमिति मन्यते।
> किमसौ मननादेव मुक्तो भवति तत्क्षणात्॥
> पुमान् जन्मान्तरशतैर्योगेनैव मुच्यते॥
>
> "After practising discrimination of the Ātman and the non-Ātman, one meditates for a long time on the fact that one is liberated on acquiring knowledge. Will he become immediately liberated by such meditation alone? No. Even after many births, he becomes liberated from bondage only through Yoga."

for,

> योगहीनं कथं ज्ञानं मोक्षदं भवतीश्वरि!।
>
> "O Goddess! How could knowledge without the method of Yoga lead to liberation?"

Thus making the point (as if it really required to be made) that theoretical knowledge and speculation without practical and direct experience is tantamount to nothing. The greatness of Yoga is likewise declared by the Bhagavadgītā:

> तपस्विभ्योऽधिको योगी ज्ञानिभ्योऽपि मतोऽधिकः।
> कर्मिभ्यश्चाधिको योगी तस्माद्योगी भवार्जुन॥ (6, 46)
>
> "The Yogin is greater than the ascetics; he is greater than even the wise or Jñānin (ज्ञानिभ्योऽपि मतोऽधिकः); he is greater than a man or action or rituals; become thou a Yogin, O Arjuna!"

We can see that even with regard to things pertaining to our ordinary life what we call knowledge is never enough, even if we are fortunate to have the right and complete kind of knowledge. This has to be made practical; it has to become an integral part of our experience. All the sophisticated calculations and theoretical knowledge required to place a man on the Moon would have been totally useless without the subsequent proper application and practical know-how of that knowledge. Knowledge is a thing of the mind; Yoga also is a thing of the mind, but a much 'deeper thing': a mind deep in Ātman. Hence, it has been written in Yājñavalkya-smṛti:

इज्याचारदमाहिंसादानस्वाध्यायकर्मणाम् ।
अयं तु परमो धर्मो यद्योगेनाऽत्मसाधनम् ॥

"Among sacrifices, customs, restraint of the senses, harmlessness, charity and Vedāntic practice, the most important is the realization of the Ātman through Yoga."

Thus indicating the pathway to Ātman, knowing which all else is known. For, there must come a time when the mind, sick, tired and exhausted of searching, becomes completely silent and calm, yet intensely one-pointed, seeking nothing for itself, absorbed in the Real Self. The following texts make this abundantly clear:

आत्मप्रयत्नसापेक्षा विशिष्टा या मनोगतिः ।
तस्या ब्रह्मणि संयोगो योग इत्यभिधीयते ॥

(*Viṣṇu Purāṇa*)

"That mental inclination which is accompanied by an intense desire to know the Self and which leads to union with the Supreme, is called Yoga."

पुरुषस्यात्यन्तिकस्वरूपावस्थितेर्हेतुश्चित्तवृत्तिनिरोधो योग इति ।

(*Yoga-sāra-saṅgraha*)

"The silencing of all mental transformations which leads to the total realization of the Supreme Self is called Yoga."

आत्मज्ञानेन मुक्तिस्स्यात् तच्च योगादृते नहि ॥

(*Skanda Purāṇa*)

"Through the knowledge of Ātman is had salvation, and that knowledge is not possible without Yoga."

योगात् संजायते ज्ञानं योगो मय्येकचित्तता ॥

(*Āditya Purāṇa*)

"Through Yoga is born knowledge of the visualization of Ātman, and Yoga is but the complete absorption of the mind in Me."

Yoga is the way to Peace, Bliss and Wisdom. In the words of the Gītā:

युञ्जन्नेवं सदाऽऽत्मानं योगी नियतमानसः ।
शान्तिं निर्वाणपरमां मत्संस्थामधिगच्छति ॥ (6, 15)

"That Yogin, with his mind controlled and poised continuously in the Ātman, attains that Peace, the Supreme Bliss that is in Me."

When, after many lives, our many desires become one final, all-consuming desire, perfectly single in its aspiration to embrace the Self, one consuming powerful flame—so to speak—forever pointing upwards, it means we have managed to 'kindle' Yoga; it is then, as Kūrma Purāṇa puts it, that:

योगाग्निर्दहति क्षिप्रमशेषपापपञ्जरम् ।
प्रसन्नं जायते ज्ञानं ज्ञानाग्निर्वाणमृच्छति ॥

"The fire of Yoga quickly consumes the entire heap of sins; thereby dawns pure knowledge, and through that knowledge, one attains salvation."

Needless to say, this is Pure Knowledge or Experience of the Self, nothing less.

What, then, is Yoga?

ऐक्यं जीवात्मनोराहुर्योगं योगविशारदाः ॥

(*Devībhāgavata*)

"Yoga adepts declare that Yoga is the union of the Jīvātman or the individual soul and Paramātman or the Supreme Soul."

संयोगो योग इत्युक्तो जीवात्मपरमात्मनोः ॥

(*Yājñavalkya-saṃhitā*)

"What is termed Yoga is the merger of the Jīvātman, the individual soul and Paramātman, the Supreme Soul."

Although, truly speaking, there is only one path or Yoga to Reality, Yoga takes many different names along the way. Many are also the 'styles' of walking or treading the path, according to the individual Sādhaka. Hence the talk about innumerable Yogas which very often throw the mind of the aspirant into confusion and disarray. The Yoga tradition is rich and colourful. To give ourselves an idea, we shall describe, if only briefly, the contents of three of the principal Yoga Upaniṣads.

Perhaps one of the richest in offering specific techniques of realization is the Dhyāna-bindu Upaniṣad. It begins with a description of the syllable OM, which every Sādhaka considers to be equivalent or identical to Brahman. The mystical syllable is praised as follows:

तैलधारामिवाच्छिन्नं दीर्घघण्टानिनादवत् ।
अवाच्यं प्रणवस्याग्रं यस्तं वेद स वेदवित् ॥

"He knows the Vedas who knows the Nāda or sound of the Praṇava OM, that is indescribable and uninterruptedly flowing like oil, just as the continuous sound of a bell that is heard even after the ringing has ceased."

In this Upaniṣad, each of the letters (a, u, m) is given a mystical colour and corresponds to a particular deity. Prāṇāyāma is identified with the three principal divinities of Vedic tradition (Brahman is said to correspond to the process of inspiration, Viṣṇu, to the process of retention or suspension, and Rudra, to the process of expiration of the breath or prāṇa). The mystical mechanism of Suṣumṇā, Iḍā and Piṅgalā, is also referred to. There is a description of the four main Āsanas, the seven Cakras and the ten principal Nāḍīs of man's subtle anatomy. It also mentions the awakening of Kuṇḍalinī. It contains the usual blinds in its description of Khecarī-mudrā, Yoni-mudrā and Bindu, which most commentators (to a large extent literalists) have been inclined to interpret in a purely sexual sense and, therefore, have surrounded the truths of Yoga by an almost impenetrable erotic mist, far, far remote from the true mysticism the text is intended to convey to the pure and enlightened Sādhaka.

The Yoga-tattva Upaniṣad mentions eight 'aṅga' or limbs and also distinguishes four types of Yoga (Mantra, Haṭha, Laya and Rāja). It lists the four principal Āsanas (Siddha, Padma, Siṃha and Bhadra). It also notes the various obstacles encountered by most Sādhakas, such as laziness, etc. The Upaniṣad mentions and describes the Prāṇāyāma technique (incorporating the usual blinds), purification of the Nāḍīs with its various accompanying signs such as clarity of pigmentation, lightness, increase in gastric power, etc. It describes some of the Siddhis, such as levitation, reading people's minds. It is said that by means of such practices the Yogin becomes very strong and beautiful, like a god; he becomes immensely attractive to members of his opposite sex; warning is given that he ought to remain forever chaste; an odour of sanctity seems to envelop him. The treatise contains a long list of Siddhis or accomplishments, i.e. invisibility, dematerialization and rematerialization, alchemy or transmutation of base metals into gold, etc. It is very rich in occult physiology connected with the various yogic disciplines. The five cosmic elements (earth, water, fire, air and ether) are described, together with the corresponding Bīja-mantras, or words of power, respective deity, for purposes of concentration and meditation.

Samādhi is described as the realization of the intrinsic unity of Jīvātman (individual soul) and Paramātman (Supreme Soul); the Yogin may subsequently seek absorption in Parabrahman or he may indeed become a god. The text is eminently practical, a kind of technical manual for the proper use of intelligent Yoga practitioners. Like all true Yoga treatises, it pursues the total spiritualization of man, immortality and liberation.

The Nāda-bindu Upaniṣad provides a very comprehensive description of what may be described as the Yoga of Sound, since the various yogic experiences are defined in terms of musical sounds and subtle vibrations, ranging from the sound of a thunderstorm, to waterfalls, the ocean, a swarm of bees, cymbals, and many other sounds of increasing degree of subtlety. Absorption in such sounds, it is said, allows the Yogin to become, eventually, totally and permanently absorbed in the inner Reality, the Ātman, which manifests at the end of all the various mystical experiences, when all sounds have subsided in the presence of the Real.

Śaṅkarācārya, in his Yoga-tārāvalī, calls this type of absorption Nādānusandhāna, and he praises it as follows:

नादानुसन्धान नमोऽस्तु तुभ्यं
त्वां मन्महे मान्यतमं लयानाम् ।
भवत्प्रसादात् पवनेन साकं
विलीयते विष्णुपदे मनो मे ॥

"O process of incessantly hearing Nāda! I bow down to you. I consider you as the worthiest of all the means for the absorption of the mind. For, through your Grace, my mind along with the vital breath gets absorbed in Viṣṇu-pada, i.e. the sky which is that Absolute Supreme of the nature of Sac-cid-ānanda."

It is the Yoga of some mediaeval saints of northern India such as Kabir, where it is referred to as Surati-śabda-yoga. This is a favourite also with the modern Rādhāsvāmī sect, the Yoga of the Sound Current, which leads to the vision and experience of the Self. To describe it in the words of Nāda-bindu Upaniṣad:

सिद्धासनस्थितो योगी मुद्रां सन्धाय वैष्णवीम् ।
शृणुयाद्दक्षिणे कर्णे नादमन्तर्गतं सदा ॥
अभ्यस्यमानो नादोऽयं बाह्यमावृणुते ध्वनिम् ।
पक्षाद्विपक्षमखिलं जित्वा तुर्यपदं व्रजेत् ॥
श्रूयते प्रथमाभ्यासे नादो नानाविधो महान् ।
वर्धमानस्तथाऽभ्यासे श्रूयते सूक्ष्मसूक्ष्मतः ॥
आदौ जलधिजीमूतभेरीनिर्झरसंभवः ।
मध्ये मर्दलशब्दाभो घण्टाकाहलजस्तथा ॥

अन्ते तु किङ्किणीवंशवीणाभ्रमरनिस्वनः ।
इति नानाविधा नादाः श्रूयन्ते सूक्ष्मसूक्ष्मतः ॥
महति श्रूयमाणे तु महाभेर्यादिकध्वनौ ।
तत्र सूक्ष्मं सूक्ष्मतरं नादमेव परामृशेत् ॥
घनमुत्सृज्य वा सूक्ष्मे सूक्ष्ममुत्सृज्य वा घने ।
रममाणमपि क्षिप्तं मनो नान्यत्र चालयेत् ॥
यत्र कुत्रापि वा नादे लगति प्रथमं मनः ।
तत्र तत्र स्थिरो भूत्वा तेन सार्धं विलीयते ॥
विस्मृत्य सकलं बाह्यं नादे दुग्धाम्बुवन्मनः ।
एकीभूयाथ सहसा चिदाकाशे विलीयते ॥
उदासीनस्ततो भूत्वा सदाऽभ्यासेन संयमी ।
उन्मनीकारकं सद्यो नादमेवावधारयेत् ॥
सर्वचिन्तां समुत्सृज्य सर्वचेष्टाविवर्जितः ।
नादमेवानुसन्दध्यान्नादे चित्तं विलीयते ॥ (31, 41)

"Seated in the posture of attainment, adopting the gesture of the pervader (Vaiṣṇavī-mudrā) with eyes wide open and without twinkling, the Yogin should continuously listen to the inner sound with the right ear. This sound, with constant practice, will drown all outer sounds. Aided by his own efforts, he conquers the external world and reaches the fourth stage. Many loud sounds are heard at first but, with practice, more and more subtle sounds are experienced. At first such sounds are like those produced by the ocean, or by a cloud, a drum, a waterfall; later, like the sound of a small drum, that of a bell, or of a musical instrument; finally, it becomes like the tinkling of bells, a flute, a lute or a bee.

Thus the many sounds are heard growing in subtlety. Even when loud sounds are heard, like those of a big drum, the Yogin should keep listening to the subtler ones. The mind should not be allowed to abandon the louder sounds for the subtler ones, or the subtler for the louder, even if it results pleasant. It should direct itself to the sound which pleased it first and become absorbed in it. So

> absorbed, the mind forgets external things and dissolves in that sound, as milk dissolves in water, to finally dissolve within the ether of consciousness. The Yogin, by constant practice, with controlled mind, becomes oblivious of everything else, and through such sounds becomes transported beyond the mind. Abandoning all thoughts and efforts, meditating on sound alone, his mind melts into sound."

It is important to note that the order of sequence in which the various sounds appear may be different according to the respective Sādhakas. It is this which makes Yoga a truly personal experimental science of Self-realization. This is our experience. The Supreme Power in manifestation, the Sacred Word OM praised in all the Vedas is capable of taking many forms. To quote from the Devī Upaniṣad:

एकैव सर्वत्र वर्तते तस्मादुच्यत एका
एकैव विश्वरूपिणी तस्मादुच्यतेऽनेका
यस्याः परतरं नास्ति ॥

"Verily the One Power pervades everywhere. Hence, it is called 'Ekā' or One (without a second).
That very Power assumes infinite forms. Hence, it is called 'Anekā' or many. Nothing surpasses that Power."

Man is one of the many forms that Supreme Power may take; a most perfect form, abode of the Eternal Self. In the words of Kṛṣṇa, in that most wonderful of the Lord's Songs, the Bhagavadgītā:

भूमिरापोऽनलो वायुः खं मनो बुद्धिरेव च ।
अहङ्कार इतीयं मे भिन्ना प्रकृतिरष्टधा ॥
अपरेयमितस्त्वन्यां प्रकृतिं विद्धि मे पराम् ।
जीवभूतां महाबाहो ययेदं धार्यते जगत् ॥ (7. 4, 5)

"Earth, water, fire, air, ether, mind, intellect and egoism —thus my Nature is eightfold. This is my Aparā (lower aspect). O Arjuna, know my other Nature different from this, that Parā or Supreme which is the life-support of the Universe."

In which passage, the word Universe also means Man. To that Supreme Power all Yogins bow. As expressed in the Devī-gītā:

नमो विराट्स्वरूपिण्यै नमः सूत्रात्ममूर्तये ।
नमोऽव्याकृतरूपिण्यै नमः श्रीब्रह्ममूर्तये ॥
नमः प्रणवरूपायै नमो ह्रींकारमूर्तये ।
सच्चिदानन्दरूपां तां गायत्रीप्रतिपादितां
नमामि नुमस्तत्पदलक्ष्यार्थम् ॥

"I bow down to that Power of the form of Virāj. I bow down to that Power that supports the entire Universe in the form of a string that runs through all. To that very Power that is unmanifest before creation I bow down. I bow down to that very Power that is of the form of the blessed Brahman. I bow down to that Power of the form of the syllable OM, of the syllable Hrīṃ. I bow down to that Power of the form of Sat (Reality) Cit (Consciousness or Energy) and Ānanda (Bliss) expressed by Gāyatrī. I praise that Power revealed by the letters of Gāyatrī-mantra.

This Power is also referred to as Nāda, the eternal, mystical call of the Real to the unreal, whereby man may discover his true heritage at the very root of his being. Such Power manifests itself in every human heart as the 'unstruck' sound. Hence, we find written in Prabodhasudhākara:

नादाभ्यन्तरवर्तिज्योतिर्यद्वर्तते हि चिरम् ।
तत्र मनो लीनं चेन्न पुनस्संसारबन्धनाय ॥

"Within the Nāda or sound is a lustre. When the mind gets absorbed in it, worldly bondage ceases."

This lustre is the radiance of the Eternal Self. Such Power plays a vital rôle in the life of the Yogin. It is at that fountain or ocean of Eternal Life that he drinks and drinks. As mystically described in the Tantras:

> पीत्वा पीत्वा पुनः पीत्वा पीत्वा पतति भूतले ।
> उत्थाय च पुनः पीत्वा पुनर्जन्म न विद्यते ॥

"Drinking and drinking, and again drinking and drinking, he falls onto the earth, but rising again and again, and drinking again and again, he knows no rebirth."

Implying something of the relentless tenacity of purpose required by the Sādhaka. The yogic path is one of total devotion, indomitable will and continuous application in the pursuit of Truth.

Modern Haṭha-yoga Tradition

The so-called modern Haṭha-yoga tradition is linked to the name Gorakhanātha, the founder of the Order of Kanphaṭā-yogins, historically placed by most authorities in the 12th century A.D., or sometimes even earlier. Such a figure is reputed to have been the author of a treatise, now lost, entitled Haṭha-yoga, and also of a preserved text which goes by the name Gorakṣaśataka. The three most well-known Haṭha-yoga 'classics', very similar in their approach (allowing for some minor differences) are:

Haṭhayoga-pradīpikā of Svātmārāma Svāmī, probably belonging to 15th century.

Śiva-saṃhitā, the longest of the three and slightly more philosophical in its approach, somewhat coloured by the Vedānta school.

Gheraṇḍa-saṃhitā, by a Vaiṣṇava from Bengal, as thought by most authorities. This is the basis of the present work and which commentary will be found, on examination, to throw a flood of light on the other two treatises.

The Yoga of the Gheraṇḍa-saṃhitā is a complete Yoga-system. It is not simply Haṭha-yoga, as this has come to be understood by innumerable 'authorities', by their failure to see things whole. It is only a mind which is becoming progressively clarified that begins to see the wholeness and interrelatedness of things.

The inability to apply a pure mind to treatises such as the one presented here is what has caused so much confusion, what has caused the Sacred Science of Yoga to be grossly misinterpreted to the point of falling into disrepute, especially in the West.

This Yoga is sevenfold. It starts with Purification leading to Strength, followed by Steadfastness and Tranquillity, followed by Lightness or Elevation, and giving rise to unveiled Spiritual Perception and perfect Liberation and Self-Realization. Its goal is Divine Wisdom or Tattva-jñāna. There is no ambiguity. The only purpose is to travel the Royal Road. As mentioned at the very beginning of the treatise: "It stands out as a ladder for those who aspire to reach the sublime heights of Rāja-yoga." It is, however, true that to the ill-informed student of Yoga it looks more like a maze than a ladder.

The Gorakṣa-saṃhitā also clearly states that:

....हठयोगविद्या विराजते प्रोन्नतराजयोगमारोढुमिच्छो-
रधिरोहिणीव ।

"The science of Haṭha-yoga is the ladder up which those climb who aspire to reach the higher regions of the Royal Path."

And the Śiva-saṃhitā, in acknowledging four stages of Yoga and in giving their progressive order according to the degree of initiation, claims:

मन्त्रयोगो हठश्चैव लययोगस्तृतीयकः ।
चतुर्थो राजयोगः स्यात्स द्विधाभाववर्जितः ॥ (5, 14)

"There are four Yogas: Mantra, Haṭha, Laya and the fourth, Rāja-yoga in which no duality remains."

And, to quote from the Haṭha-yoga-pradīpikā:

केवलं राजयोगाय हठविद्योपदिश्यते । (1, 2)

"For the sake of Rāja-yoga alone is Haṭha-yoga taught."

Thus clarifying motive and purpose beyond the shadow of a doubt.

PURIFICATIONS

Because of the technical nature of treatises such as the present one, the mistake is often made in thinking that the need for Purification is limited to the Ṣaṭkarma-s, since these are the only physical purificatory acts or requirements mentioned by Gheraṇḍa. This has led people to think, rather wrongly, that the Yoga of the Gheraṇḍa-saṃhitā is somehow inferior to other Yogas, i.e. Bhakti-yoga, Jñāna-yoga, Karma-yoga, Rāja-yoga, and so on. The truth of the matter is that, in attempting to bring the body and mind to its highest peak of health and efficiency, the question of moral qualifications, or fitness for discipleship, is not ignored, but rather taken for granted by the wise Gheraṇḍa. The Sādhaka requires to be ten times more disciplined and dedicated than a participant in the Olympic Games, if he is to succeed. Therefore, a solid if not altogether perfect, ethical foundation is a must. His is the game of Eternal Life and Perfect Liberation.

Such moral qualifications one finds variously described in many places. Patañjali-yoga-sūtras, for example, refer to these as Yamas or abstinences:

अहिंसासत्यास्तेयब्रह्मचर्यापरिग्रहा यमाः । (2, 30)

"Non-violence, truth, non-stealing, chastity and non-possessiveness."

and Niyamas or observances:

शौचसन्तोषतपःस्वाध्यायेश्वरप्रणिधानानि नियमाः । (2, 32)

"Purity, contentment, austerity, self-development and constant thought of the Divine."

The value and importance of such ethical requirements is not to be neglected or underestimated, for, these moral qualifications, when in full bloom or developed to perfection, can even manifest as spiritual powers of a very high order, nay, they constitute a gateway to the Immortal Self. So, in the same Yoga-sūtras, we read:

अपरिग्रहस्थैर्ये जन्मकथन्तासम्बोधः । (2, 39)

"When non-possessiveness is firmly established there arises knowledge of the mystery of births."

and,

सत्त्वशुद्धिसौमनस्यैकाग्र्येन्द्रियजयात्मदर्शनयोग्यत्वानि च ।
(2, 41)

"By purity, the mind becomes happy and concentrated, capable of witnessing the Self."

Of such ethical foundations, the Viṣṇu Purāṇa also speaks in glowing terms:

एते यमास्सनियमाः पञ्च पञ्च च कीर्तिताः ।
विशिष्टफलदाः काम्या निष्कामाणां विमुक्तिदाः ॥ (6, 7, 38)

"The abstinences and observances each number five; by practising them with their given purpose in mind, they yield such results; by practising without desire, they lead to liberation."

Thus also giving a hint on the overall important question of motive. The Yoga-śikhā Upaniṣad also praises in unmistakable terms the merits of a truly spiritual life as the perfect foundation of the perfect Yogin, as can be clearly seen in the following passage:

कामक्रोधभयं चापि मोहलोभमयो रमः ।
जन्म मृत्युश्च कार्पण्यं शोकस्तन्द्रा क्षुधा तृषा ॥
तृष्णा लज्जा भयं दुखं विषादो हर्ष एव च ।
एभिर्दोषैर्विनिर्मुक्तः स जीवः शिव उच्यते ॥ (10-11)

"He who is free from lust, anger, fear, error, greed, passion, birth, death, cupidity, melancholy, laziness, hunger, thirst, desire, shyness, pain, temper, and extreme gladness is called Śiva."

The impression has often been given that Haṭha-yoga is all about extreme asceticism and formidable practices, physical rigour and bodily and mental prowess; whereas, in fact, Haṭha-yoga is all about common sense and the avoidance of extremes of any kind; it seeks the 'middle' way, the centre of things; it aims for that 'holy land' which lies beyond the pairs of opposites, beyond heat and cold, in-breathing, and out-breathing, self and not-self. Has it not been rightly said by Kṛṣṇa in the Gītā:

> नात्यश्नतस्तु योगोऽस्ति न चैकान्तमनश्नतः ।
> न चातिस्वप्नशीलस्य जाग्रतो नैव चार्जुन ॥
> युक्ताहारविहारस्य युक्तचेष्टस्य कर्मसु ।
> युक्तस्वप्नावबोधस्य योगो भवति दुःखहा ॥ (6, 16-17)

> "O Arjuna, this yoga is not attained by him who overeats, nor by him who fasts. Nor by him who oversleeps, nor by him who keeps awake.
> This yoga which banishes pain is attained by him who eats and behaves properly, whose actions are led by reason, whose sleep and wake are regulated."

And in the Garuḍa Purāṇa, don't we read:

> "Donkeys move about among people, in forests and among dwellings, quite naked and unashamed. Are these free from attachment?...
> Do the crocodile, fish and others, which from birth to death dwell in the waters of the Ganges, become Yogins?..." (XVI)

The fact is often missed that the teachings of Gheraṇḍa-saṃhitā are closely interrelated, and there is more to these six purificatory practices than meets the eye. For example, under Trāṭaka (verses 53 and 54) we read:

> "Without winking, gaze steadily at any small object until tears begin to flow. The wise call this practice Trāṭaka. Success in this practice leads to Śāmbhavī-mudrā. It cures all diseases of the eyes and induces clairvoyance."

That this practice cures all diseases of the eyes may be important enough; that it induces clairvoyance may prove indeed useful; but, what is really of untold worth is that such practice leads to Śāmbhavī-mudrā. Although Yoga treatises speak of only one form of Trāṭaka, the Upaniṣads mention three different forms: the outer fixing, the intermediate fixing and the inner fixing of the gaze—in progressive stages of interiorization. The Haṭhayoga-pradīpikā describes Trāṭaka as follows:

निरीक्षेन्निश्चलदृशा सूक्ष्मलक्ष्यं समाहितः ।
अश्रुसम्पातपर्यन्तमाचार्यैस्त्राटकं स्मृतम् ॥ (2, 31)

"Fixing intently the sight, without winking, on a minute object until tears come to the eyes is known to the Great Teachers as Trāṭaka."

And Gorakṣa-saṃhitā also describes it in a similar manner (2, 9).

The Maṇḍala-brāhmaṇa Upaniṣad, in referring to Yoga, states:

तद्योगं च द्विविधा विद्धि पूर्वोत्तरविभागतः
पूर्वं तु तारकं विद्यादमनस्कं तदुत्तरम् ॥
भ्रूयुगमध्यबिले तेजस आविर्भावः एतत् पूर्वतारकं ।
उत्तरं त्वमनस्कम् ॥
तद्दर्शने तिस्रो दृष्टयः अमा प्रतिपत् पूर्णिमा चेति ॥

"Know that Yoga is of two kinds, earlier and later. The earlier is known as Tāraka, and the later as Amanaska.
When the light begins to manifest in the middle of the eyebrows, that is called Tāraka; when the mind is absorbed, it is Amanaska.
For its visualization, there are three ways of looking at that: (1) Amā, (2) Pratipat and (3) Pūrṇimā."

These three ways of looking are subsequently defined as follows:

"निमीलितदर्शनममादृष्टिः अर्धोन्मीलितं प्रतिपत् सर्वोन्मीलनं पूर्णिमा भवति"

"Looking with the eyes closed is Amādṛṣṭi; looking with the eyes half-closed is Pratipat-dṛṣṭi; looking with wide-opened eyes is Pūrṇimādṛṣṭi."

The last way of looking goes also by the name of Śāmbhavī-mudrā (शाम्भवीमुद्रा). It is said that if meditation at the centre of the eyebrows is practised in anyone of these three ways, Rāja-yoga can be achieved.

It is clear, then, that the ladder of Gheraṇḍa-saṃhitā, truly extends from the lowest rung to the very highest. It is therefore a mistake to refer to this work simply as a Haṭha-yoga treatise.

Āsanas

After describing the basic purificatory practices, Gheraṇḍa goes on to describe the postures or Āsanas, producers of strength, conducive to good health and preliminary to Steadfastness in Yoga, as signified by the Mudrās—the latter being the inner side of the Āsana.

The Gheraṇḍa-saṃhitā mentions 32 Āsanas with some of the benefits derived from them. A different number of postures is given in detail by different books on Yoga; for example, the Haṭha-yoga-pradīpikā describes 14; the Yogapradīpa, 21; the Viśva-kośa, 32; the Anubhava-prakāśa, 50. However, they all seem to agree that the number of chief postures is 84, allowing, of course, for certain minor technical differences among them. Four of these postures are very generally practised and favoured by yogins: Siddhāsana, Padmāsana, Svastikāsana and Siṃhāsana.

It has been said in the Triśikhī Upaniṣad:

आसनं विजितं येन जितं तेन जगत्त्रयम् । (52)

"He who masters the postures conquers the three worlds."

In the Bhagavadgītā, Kṛṣṇa prescribes the Āsana as follows:

शुचौ देशे प्रतिष्ठाप्य स्थिरमासनमात्मन: ।
नात्युच्छ्रितं नातिनीचं चैलाजिनकुशोत्तरम् ।।
तत्रैकाग्रं मन: कृत्वा यतचित्तेन्द्रियक्रिय: ।
उपविश्यासने युञ्ज्याद्योगमात्मविशुद्धये ।।

समं कायशिरोग्रीवं धारयन्नचलं स्थिरः ।
संप्रेक्ष्य नासिकाग्रं स्वं दिशश्चानवलोकयन् ॥
प्रशान्तात्मा विगतभीर्ब्रह्मचारिव्रते स्थितः ।
मनः संयम्य मच्चित्तो युक्त आसीत मत्परः ॥ (6, 11-14)

"In a pure spot, on a firm seat neither too high nor too low made of a cloth, deer skin and kuśa grass, there, with the senses subdued, the mind one-pointed and free of thoughts, he should practise Yoga for the purpose of purification. Holding the body, head and neck aligned, perfectly steady, gazing at the end of the nose yet not seeing, serene, fearless, harmonized, with mind absorbed in Me, let him sit aspiring towards Me."

A much similar injunction is given in the Bhāgavata Purāṇa, Chapter 14.

Mudrās

Generally speaking, the word Mudrā is used to signify certain postures, contractions, gestures and positions of hands and fingers (such as Padma-mudrā or symbol of the Lotus and Yoni-liṅga-mudrā or symbol of ecstatic union) of varied use to the yogin in the manipulation of Prāṇa and other subtle energies.

Mudrās occupy a central place in the Yoga of Gheraṇḍa-saṃhitā, and under the somewhat formidable and dramatic 'material' descriptions there lies a mine of spiritual treasures awaiting to be discovered by the intelligent Sādhaka. They combine all the elements of Yoga practice, i.e. mastery of posture, mastery of breath and inner processes, perfect concentration and meditation to the end of Samādhi. Gheraṇḍa-saṃhitā is particularly rich in this respect, describing in detail 26 of them. Although many are the Mudrās utilized in Yoga practice, basically all systems include at least the three vital contractions known as Mūla-bandha (Root-contraction), Uḍḍīyāna-bandha (Flying-up-contraction) and Jālandhara-bandha (Chin-contraction or lock). The Śiva-saṃhitā, for example, gives only ten prominent Mudrās, as follows: Mahā-mudrā, Mahā-bandha, Mahā-vedha, Khecarī, Viparīta-karaṇī, Vajrolī, Śakti-cālanī,

Mūla-bandha, Jālandhara-bandha and Uḍḍīyāna-bandha. The Mudrā system relates to a very sophisticated, delicate and subtle network of interflowing energies. Its purpose is to 'awaken' Divinity. In the words of Śiva-saṃhitā:

सुप्ता गुरुप्रसादेन यदा जार्गात कुण्डली ।
तदा सर्वाणि पद्मानि भिद्यन्ते ग्रन्थयोऽपि च ।।
तस्मात् सर्वप्रयत्नेन प्रबोधयितुमीश्वरीम् ।
ब्रह्मरन्ध्रमुखे सुप्तां मुद्राभ्यासं समाचरेत् ।। (4, 22-23)

"Helped by the Guru, after the sleeping coiled energy has awakened and pierced all the subtle centres and their knots, then, in order to awaken the Divine sleeping in Brahmarandhra, the Mudrās should be practised intensively."

Two Mudrās are of particular importance for the awakening of the Divine, the Śāmbhavī-mudrā and the Khecarī-mudrā. The former has been described in Haṭha-yoga-pradīpikā as follows:

अन्तर्लक्ष्यं बहिर्दृष्टिर्निमेषोन्मेषवर्जिता ।
एषा सा शाम्भवीमुद्रा सर्वतन्त्रेषु गोपिता ।।

"The mind is to be concentrated on anyone of the subtle centres from Mūlādhāra onwards to Brahmarandhra. Externally, the eye is to be fixed in a gaze without winking. This is that well-known Śāmbhavī-mudrā, and it is kept secret in all Tantras."

Khecarī-mudrā is generally taken to mean the swallowing of the tongue. The Dhyāna-bindu Upaniṣad describes it as follows:

न पीयूषं पतत्यग्नौ न च वायु: प्रयावति ।
कपालकुहरे जिह्वा प्रविष्टा विपरीतगा ।।
भ्रुवोरन्तर्गता दृष्टिर्मुद्रा भवति खेचरी । (79-80)

"The nectar (from the thousand-petalled lotus) no longer flows into the fire (of the stomach) nor does the vital-breath go out when the backward-turned tongue enters the cranial cavity (behind the glottis). If the gaze is then fixed between the eye-brows, this is known as Khecarī-(moving in the Void) mudrā or gesture."

The same Upaniṣad praises Khecarī in the following words, full of mystical symbolism:

खेचर्या मुद्रया यस्य विवरं लम्बिकोर्ध्वतः ।
बिन्दुः क्षरति नो यस्य कामिन्यालिङ्गितस्य च ॥
यावद् बिन्दुः स्थितो देहे तावन्मृत्युभयं कुतः ।
यावद् बद्धा नभोमुद्रा तावद् बिन्दुर्न गच्छति ॥
गलितोऽपि यदा बिन्दुः सम्प्राप्तो योनिमण्डले ।
व्रजत्यूर्ध्वं हठाच्छक्त्या निबद्धो योनिमुद्रया । (83-86)

"He who practises Khecarī, with tongue in the hole above the glottis, and whose seed does not flow even when embraced by a woman, who preserves his seed, what fear has he of death? The seed cannot fall so long as the gesture of the Void is held. Even if the seed happened to fall, then, on reaching the womb, it is drawn up again by virtue of Yoni-mudrā."

This 'drawing-up again' is known as Vajrolī-mudrā, to be understood not literally and in erotic terms but esoterically, in terms of a mystical marriage: The Śiva-śakti 'embrace'!

The process is rightly understood by the writer of Maṇḍala-brāhmaṇa Upaniṣad, when he acknowledges that.

एवं सहजानन्दे यदा मनो लीयते तदा शांभवी भवति ।
तामेव खेचरीमाहुः ॥ (2, 18)

"When the mind dissolves into its inherent bliss, this is the gesture of the Giver of Happiness. This is also called the Moving-in-the-Void gesture."

That Khecarī-mudrā is meant to be understood mystically, as referring to the vivid flame or tongue of fire arising within the yogin's subtle anatomy, can be deduced from one of those very few unguarded remarks contained in Yoga literature, in this case the Śiva-saṃhitā:

इह नाडी नदी प्रोक्ता शरीरे वर्तते सदा ।
पवनस्य गतिस्तत्र सर्वतः स्नानमुच्यते ॥
'सुषुम्नैव परं तीर्थं' सुषुम्नैव परा गतिः ॥

"Here, in the body, there is always a river, the Suṣumnā nerve. The passing of the vital breath through that nerve is what is called Snāna or holy bath. Suṣumnā is verily the most sacred place of pilgrimage. Suṣumnā is verily the ultimate goal."

All the Cakras are 'threaded' by the subtlest of the subtlest: Suṣumnā! These Cakras have distinct forms and colours which can be clearly perceived by the yogin, especially when the system has been activated by the awakening and subsequent rising of Kuṇḍalinī-śakti, the ever-creative, evolutionary and redemptive Supreme Power which abides in every individual and which permeates all things. Descriptions of these centres vary slightly according to the respective 'schools' of Yoga. Such differences, however, are in most instances minor and superficial. They combine clairvoyant visualization with mystic symbolism, form, colour and sound (corresponding to the letters of the Sanskrit alphabet), and a host of deities in charge of the various centres or lotuses.

Such descriptions provide a highly 'structural' approach and ought not to be taken always too literally. It may be useful to some of our readers—as complementary to the instructions given by Gheraṇḍa—if we here describe some of the aspects of the Cakras as found in the Śiva-saṃhitā. Starting with the centre situated at the base of the spine:

Mūlādhāra Cakra

आधारपद्ममेतद्धि योनिर्यस्यास्ति कन्दतः ।
परिस्फुरत् वादिसान्तचतुर्वर्णं चतुर्दलम् ॥ (5, 83)
कुलाभिधं सुवर्णाभं स्वयम्भूलिङ्गसङ्गतम् ।
द्विरण्डो यत्र सिद्धोऽस्ति डाकिनी यत्र देवता ॥
तत्पद्ममध्यमा योनिस्तत्र कुण्डलिनी स्थिता ।
तस्या ऊर्ध्वे स्फुरत्तेजः कामबीजं भ्रमन्मतम् ॥

यः करोति सदा ध्यानं मूलाधारे विचक्षणः ।
तस्य स्याद्दार्दुरी सिद्धिर्भूमित्यागक्रमेण वै ॥ (5, 84-86)

"This is the root-lotus of which the Yoni is the heart. The centre is most brilliant, with four petals bearing the four letters v, ś, ṣ, s."

This centre is known as Kula (womb) and shines like gold; here is found the Svayambhū-liṅga or symbol of the Self-born. Here is found the Realized Being (Siddha) named Double-edged (Dviraṇḍa). The host deity of this centre is Dākinī. In the middle of the lotus is the Yoni, and in it the coiled-up energy. Just above it, the shining seed of Passion (Kāma-bīja) wanders like a flame. The wise man who ever meditates on this centre realizes the Frog (Dārdurī), the faculty of wandering through space."

Svādhiṣṭhāna Cakra

द्वितीयन्तु सरोजं च लिङ्गमूले व्यवस्थितम् ।
बादिलान्तं च षड्वर्णं परिभास्वरषड्दलम् ॥
स्वाधिष्ठानाभिधं तत्तु पङ्कजं शोणरूपकम् ।
बाणाख्यो यत्र सिद्धोऽस्ति देवो यत्रास्ति राकिणी ॥ (5, 98-99)

"The second centre named 'support of the life-breath' lies at the root of the penis (white in colour) and it has six red petals bearing the letters b, bh, m, y, r, l. Here abides the Realized Being called Arrow (Bāṇa). The host deity is Rākiṇī."

Maṇipūra Cakra

तृतीयं पङ्कजं नाभौ मणिपूरकसंज्ञकम् ।
दशारण्डादिफान्तार्णं शोभितं हेमवर्णकम् ॥
रुद्राख्यो यत्र सिद्धोऽस्ति सर्वमङ्गलदायकः ।
तत्रस्था लाकिनीनाम्नी देवी परमधार्मिका ॥ (5, 104-105)

तस्मिन् ध्यानं सदा योगी करोति मणिपूरके ।
तस्य पातालसिद्धिः स्यान्निरन्तरसुखावहा ॥

ईप्सितं च भवेल्लोके दुःखरोगविनाशनम् ।
कालस्य वञ्चनं चापि परदेहप्रवेशनम् ॥
जाम्बूनदादिकरणं सिद्धानां दर्शनं भवेत् ।
ओषधीदर्शनं चापि निधीनां दर्शनं भवेत् ॥ (5, 106-108)

"The third centre, the Jewel-city (Maṇipūra) is situated in the region of the navel. It has ten golden petals bearing the letters ḍ, ḍh, ṇ, t, th, d, dh, n, p and ph. Here abides the Realized Being, provider of boons, named Rudra. The host deity of the centre is the supremely virtuous Goddess Lākinī."

He who ever meditates on this Maṇipūra Cakra gains the Pātāla attainment, giver of all other attainments. Disease and pain are destroyed, all desires are fulfilled and Time is vanquished, and the seeker can enter into other people's bodies. He acquires the gift of making gold and other precious substances. He knows medicinal plants and can unveil treasures."

Anāhata Cakra

हृदयेऽनाहतं नाम चतुर्थं पङ्कजं भवेत् ।
कादिठान्तार्णसंस्थानं द्वादशारसमन्वितम् ॥
अतिशोणं वायुबीजं प्रसादस्थानमीरितम् । (5, 109)
ज्ञानं चाप्रतिमं तस्य त्रिकालविषयं भवेत् ।
दूरश्रुतिर्दूरदृष्टिः स्वेच्छया खगतां व्रजेत् ॥ (5, 112)

"The fourth lotus is in the heart; it is named the centre of unstruck sound (Anāhata). It has twelve petals of flaming red bearing the letters k, kh, g, gh, ṅ, c, ch, j, jh, ñ, ṭ, and ṭh. Here dwells in delight the Seed of Wind (Vāyu-bīja); it is the source of the vital breath."

"Supramental knowledge arises in the seeker's mind. He sees past, present and future; he is capable of hearing from afar and perceives subtle and distant things. At will, he can wander through space."

Viśuddha Cakra

कण्ठस्थानस्थितं पत्रं विशुद्धं नाम पञ्चमम् ।
सुहेमाभं स्वरोपेतं षोडशस्वरसंयुतम् ॥
छगलाण्डोऽस्ति सिद्धोऽत्र शाकिनी चाधिदेवता । (5, 116)
ध्यानं करोति यो नित्यं स योगीश्वरपण्डितः ।
किन्त्वस्य योगिनोऽन्यत्र विशुद्धाख्ये सरोरुहे ॥
चतुर्वेदा विभासन्ते सरहस्या निधेरिव । (5, 117)

"The fifth lotus is in the throat; it is known as the centre of Great Purity; it glows like good gold (others say smoke-coloured). It has sixteen petals bearing the vowels a, ā, i, ī, u, ū, ṛ, ṝ, ḷ, ḹ, e, ai, o, au, aṃ, aḥ. Here is the Realized Being named Chagalāṇḍa (the goat's egg). The host deity is the Goddess Śākinī (the leafed)."

"He who concentrates on this centre becomes a master of the Sacred Wisdom and a prince amongst yogins. In this lotus of Great Purity, he contemplates the four Scriptures of Eternal Wisdom (The Vedas) like a bountiful ocean full of secret meanings."

Ājñā Cakra

आज्ञापद्मं भ्रुवोर्मध्ये हक्षोपेतं द्विपत्रकम् ।
शुक्लाभं तन्महाकालः सिद्धो देव्यत्र हाकिनी ॥
शरच्चन्द्रनिभं तत्राक्षरबीजं विजृम्भितम् ।
पुमान् परमहंसोऽयं यज्ज्ञात्वा नावसीदति ॥
तत्र देवः परं तेजः सर्वतन्त्रेषु मन्त्रिणः ।
चिन्तयित्वा परां सिद्धिं लभते नात्र संशयः ॥ (5, 122-123)
राजयोगाधिकारी स्यादेतच्चिन्तनतो ध्रुवम् ।
योगी बन्धाद्विनिर्मुक्तः स्वीयया प्रभया स्वयम् ॥
द्विदलध्यानमाहात्म्यं कथितुं नैव शक्यते ।
ब्रह्मादिदेवताश्चैव किंचिन्मत्तो विदन्ति ते ॥ (5, 149)

"Between the eye-brows, with two petals bearing the

letters h and kṣ, is the lotus or centre of command. It is white in colour. Here abides the Realized Being named Arch-Time (Mahā-kāla). The host deity is Hākinī."

"The luminous Lunar-seed, like the Moon of the cool season, is here well established. Conscious of it, the discerning seeker is ever freed from pain. The host deity is the Supreme Light hidden in all the Tantras. Absorbed in it, he attains Supreme Realization definitely."

"The yogin who meditates on this is doubtless worthy of the Royal Road (Rāja-yoga); by his own power he frees himself from bondage. No man can ever describe the greatness of meditation on this two-petalled lotus. The Creator and all the other gods learnt something about it from Me."

Brahmarandhra or Sahasrāra Cakra

अत ऊर्ध्वं तालुमूले सहस्रारं सरोरुहम् ।
अस्ति यत्र सुषुम्नाया मूलं सविवरं स्थितम् (5, 150)
अत ऊर्ध्वं दिव्यरूपं सहस्रारं सरोरुहम् ।
ब्रह्माण्डाख्यस्य देहस्य बाह्ये तिष्ठति मुक्तिदम् ॥
कैलासो नाम तस्यैव महेशो यत्र तिष्ठति ।
अकुलाख्योऽविनाशी च क्षयवृद्धिविवर्जितः ॥ (5, 186-87)
स्थाने परे हंसनिवासभूते कैलासनाम्नीह निविष्टचेताः ।
योगी हतव्याधिरधःकृताधिर्वायुश्चिरं जीवति मृत्युमुक्तः ॥
(5, 189)

तस्माद्गलितपीयूषं पिबेद्योगी निरन्तरम् ।
मृत्योर्मृत्युं विधायाशु कुलं जित्वा सरोरुहे ॥
अत्र कुण्डलिनी शक्तिर्लयं याति कुलाभिधा ।
तदा चतुर्विधा सृष्टिर्लीयते परमात्मनि ॥ (5, 192-193)

"At the root of the palate, above the centre of command, is the lotus of a thousand petals. It is here, at the root of the Brahmarandhra, that Suṣumnā, the central nerve of the subtle body ends."

"Above the palate is the divine lotus of a thousand petals.

Giver of Liberation, it stands outside the body said to be the Universe. It is named Kailāsa where the immortal great god named Akula, devoid of decay and growth dwells."

"In this place named Kailāsa dwells the swan of Supreme Discrimination. He who fixes his mind on the thousand-petalled lotus achieves the end of all suffering. Free from death, he becomes immortal."

"The yogin continuously drinks the ambrosia flowing from this lotus. Having vanquished death and the root of Nature, he becomes immortal. It is here that the coiled-up energy, Kuṇḍalinī-śakti, also known as Womb (Kula) dissolves. The fourfold manifestation is then reabsorbed into the Supreme Being."

Pratyāhāra

Gheraṇḍa's fourth lesson has to do with emotional and mental control of the senses. According to Yājñavalkya-saṃhitā, the ideal way of achieving this is by means of a thorough and disciplined understanding of the 'ascent' and "descent" (āroha-avaroha) of the life-breath, to be gained only while living near a qualified teacher or guru. Yājñavalkya mentions 18 Ādhāras or centres of energy through which conscious withdrawal takes place. The number of centres utilized varies according to the various schools; Śiva-yoga mentions 16 Ādhāras. Elaboration on this interesting and practical topic would require many pages; suffice it to say that it forms the basis for certain very advanced Yoga techniques in which Prāṇāyāma plays a very crucial rôle.

The Viṣṇu Purāṇa refers to Pratyāhāra or the withdrawal of the senses in the following words:

शब्दाविष्वनुरक्तानि निगृह्याक्षीणि योगवित् ।
कुर्याच्चित्तानुकारीणि प्रत्याहारपरायणः ॥
वश्यता परमा तेन जायतेऽतिचलात्मनाम् ।
इन्द्रियाणामवश्यस्तैर्न योगी योगसाधकः ॥ (6, 7, 43-44)

"The successful Sādhaka faithfully practises 'withdrawal' and stops the contact of the senses with the various objects to which they are invariably attached. The ever-agitated senses are then controlled, at the service of his conscious will. No yogin can ever succeed in Yoga without sense-control."

As for the Gītā, Kṛṣṇa's advice is simple enough:

तानि सर्वाणि संयम्य युक्त आसीत मत्परः ।
वशे हि यस्येन्द्रियाणि तस्य प्रज्ञा प्रतिष्ठिता ॥ (2, 61)

"Let him restrain all the senses and, concentrating the mind, surrender to Me, for he who has his senses under control understands aright."

Only he who has perfect control of the senses enjoys profound peace and tranquillity.

Prāṇāyāma

One of the most important elements in the Yoga of Gheraṇḍa-saṃhitā, central to Yoga, is Prāṇāyāma or what is sometimes described as regulation and retention of the breath. Gheraṇḍa deals here with the question of time and place and regulated nourishment, the purification of the Nāḍīs, the various Prāṇas, Kumbhaka or Prāṇāyāma proper which is eightfold: Sahita, Sūryabheda, Ujjāyī, Śitalī, Bhastrikā, Brāhmarī, Mūrcchā and Kevalī. He also describes the ladder of mystic sounds which manifests in the invisible anatomy of the Sādhaka as his proficiency in Prāṇāyāma practice continues to develop. He sings the excellences of Kevalī based on the Ajapā Gāyatrī (Haṃsaḥ), that ineffable, non-uttered Japa forever present in all living beings. He concludes: "For him who knows Yoga, Prāṇāyāma is Kevalī. What can he not accomplish on this earth who has achieved mastery in Kevala-kumbhaka?

The importance of Prāṇāyāma (properly understood) and how great a part it plays in the correct practice of Yoga is demonstrated by the following passages. It is written in Haṭha-yoga-pradīpikā:

इन्द्रियाणां मनो नाथो मनोनाथस्तु मारुतः ।
मारुतस्य लयो नाथः स लयो नादमाश्रितः ॥ (4, 29)

"The mind is the master of the senses; the life-breath is the master of the mind; the master of the life-breath is its absorption. The absorption of the mind is achieved by (listening to) the inner sound."

The Śiva-saṃhitā, also, extols its virtues:

प्राणायामेन योगीन्द्रो लब्ध्वैश्वर्याष्टकानि च ।
पापपुण्योदधिं तीर्त्वा त्रैलोक्यचरतामियात् ॥ (3, 61)

"The Master of Yoga, through breath-control, acquires the eight superhuman powers. He crosses beyond the ocean of sin and virtue and freely wanders in the three worlds."

Śaṅkarācārya's opinion, in his commentary to Śvetāśvatara Upaniṣad, is certainly unmistakable in his praise of Prāṇāyāma:

प्राणायामविशुद्धात्मा यस्मात्पश्यति तत्परम् ॥
तस्मान्नातः परं किंचित् प्राणायामादिति श्रुतिः ॥
(Comm. on 2, 7)

"The soul purified by Prāṇāyāma realizes the Supreme Spirit (Parabrahman). Hence, according to Supreme Revelation, the Śruti, there is nothing superior to Prāṇāyāma."

In the words of Yājñavalkya-saṃhitā:

प्राणसंयमनेनैव सर्वे मुक्ता भवन्ति हि ।
प्राणायामैर्विशुद्धा ये ते यान्ति परमां गतिम् ॥
संसारार्णवमग्नानां तारकः प्राणसंयमः ॥

"All become liberated verily by the control of Prāṇa. They all attain salvation who get purified by Prāṇāyāma. The control of Prāṇa, truly, is the vessel that carries the afflicted across the ocean of manifestation to Liberation."

For Patañjali also, Prāṇāyāma plays a leading rôle, for it clears away the obstacles on the path of the Sādhaka:

ततः क्षीयते प्रकाशावरणम् । धारणासु च योग्यता मनसः ।
(2, 52-53)

"Then the veil which covers the Light is destroyed and the mind becomes capable of concentration."

And Vyāsa, commenting on the above verse, states:

तपो न परं प्राणायामात् । ततो विशुद्धिर्मलानां दीप्तिश्च ज्ञानस्य ।

"There is no discipline which leads higher than breath-control. It purifies all impurity and kindles the flame of understanding."

The Brahma-vidyā Upaniṣad describes the non-uttered (Ajapā) Japa as follows:

दृश्यं तं दिव्यरूपेण सर्वव्यापी निरञ्जनः ।
हंस हंस वदेद्वाक्यं प्राणिनां देहमाश्रितः ।
स प्राणापानयोर्ग्रन्थिरजपेत्यभिधीयते ।
सहस्रमेकं द्व्ययुतं षट्शतं चैव सर्वदा ॥
उच्चरन्पतितो हंसः सोऽहमित्यभिधीयते ॥ (78-79)

"His Divine Form, unveiled, can be seen permeating all things. 'I am He (Aham-saḥ)', the mantra of identification, abides in the body of all beings, at the place where the incoming and outgoing breaths (Prāṇa-apāna) merge. This is called the non-uttered (Ajapa) repetition of His name. Everyday, 21,600 times this utterance 'I am He, He I am' (Haṃsaḥ/So'haṃ) rises and falls (with the life-breath)."

And the Haṃsa Upaniṣad describes the ladder of mystic sounds (not to be confused, as it is often the case, with the cardio-vascular noises pertaining to the circulation of the blood) in the following words:

> चिणीति प्रथमः; चिञ्चिणीति द्वितीयः; घण्टानाद-
> स्तृतीयः; शङ्खनादश्चतुर्थः; पञ्चमस्तन्त्रीनादः;
> षष्ठस्ताळनादः; सप्तमो वेणुनादः; अष्टमो मृदङ्गनादः;
> नवमो भेरीनादः; दशमो मेघनादः ॥

> "Ciṇ is a sort of onomatopoeic sound; this is the first audible sound. The second is the sound 'Ciñ-ciṇ'. The third is like a pealing tone of a bell. The blowing sound of the conch resembles the fourth. The sound of a Vīṇā (musical instrument) is the fifth. That of Tāla (rythmic cadence) is the sixth. The seventh is like the sound of a flute, and that of a Mṛdaṅga (type of drum) the eighth. The ninth is the sound of a kettle-drum and the tenth like the rumbling of thunder of the clouds."

The Tejo-bindu Upaniṣad describes Prāṇāyāma in rather more mystical terms, as it is often the case in that treatise:

> निषेधनं प्रपञ्चस्य रेचकाख्यः समीरितः ।
> ब्रह्मैवास्मीति या वृत्तिः पूरको वायुरुच्यते ॥
> ततस्तद्वृत्तिनैश्चल्यं कुम्भकं प्राणसंयमः ।
> अयं चापि प्रबुद्धानामज्ञानां घ्राणपीडनम् ॥ (1, 32-33)

> "The conviction of the unreality of the world is called breathing out. The repeated feeling 'I am the Supreme Principle' (Brahman), is called breathing in. When this feeling is permanently fixed in the mind, it is called holding of the breath. Such is the breath-control of the wise; controlling the breath by pressing the nostrils is the way of the ignorant."

Thus endeavouring to convey that there is more to the concept or practice of Prāṇāyāma than meets the eye, and that it has little if anything to do with the 'physical' retention of the breath, as wrongly understood by the great majority of people, and as we have tried to demonstrate in our commentary on the Gheraṇḍa-saṃhitā.

For Yogacintāmaṇi the position is clear:

प्राणायाम एवाभ्यासक्रमेण वर्धमानः
प्रत्याहारधारणाध्यानसमाधिशब्दैरुच्यते ॥

"The processes of Pratyāhāra, Dhāraṇā, Dhyāna and Samādhi are truly Prāṇāyāma gradually increasing in the practice."

And the Haṭha-yoga-pradīpikā, cryptically declares that:

"ब्रह्मरन्ध्रं गतः प्राणो यदा पञ्चविंशतिपलपर्यन्तं
तिष्ठति तदा प्रत्याहारः, यदा पञ्चघटिकापर्यन्तं
तिष्ठति तदा धारणा, यदा षष्टिघटिकापर्यन्तं
तिष्ठति तदा ध्यानं, यदा द्वादशदिनपर्यन्तं
तिष्ठति तदा समाधिर्भवति" (2, 12)

"If the air that has entered the Brahmarandhra is retained there for about 25 Palas, that is Pratyāhāra. If it remains for 5 ghaṭikās (two hours), it is Dhāraṇā. If it stays for 60 ghaṭikās, it is Dhyāna. Remaining thus for 12 days it becomes Samādhi."

When properly understood, many are the excellences of Prāṇāyāma. Wrongly understood, it is entirely fruitless and, indeed, it may become even harmful.

To leave the final word with that ancient classic of untold merit, the Yoga-Vāsiṣhta:

एषा हि चितिविश्रान्तिर्मया प्राणसमाधिना ।
क्रमेणानेन संप्राप्ता स्वयमात्मनि निर्मले ॥

"Gradually, by Prāṇāyāma practice, I attained absorption of the mind in that Immaculate Supreme Ātman."

Dhyāna-yoga/samādhi

The two final lessons of Gheraṇḍa-saṃhitā deal with meditation and the end of meditation, i.e. Samādhi. In other words, with Spiritual Perception and Perfect Liberation. Three kinds of meditation are described by Gheraṇḍa: Sthūla (directed to physical objects, figures or forms), Jyotis (having for support the mysteries of the light and the substance of the inner worlds) and Sūkṣma (relating to Brahman, Ātman and Kuṇḍalinī-śakti) the sphere of influence of Śāṃbhavī and Khecarī-mudrās proper. The end of all true Yoga meditation being the attainment of Samādhi, the wise Gheraṇḍa goes on to describe six 'types' of Samādhi or stages of mental absorption in the Real (Dhyāna, Nāda, Rasānanda, Laya-siddhi, Bhakti and Rāja). And, in praising the sublimity of Samādhi, he says:

> "O Caṇḍa! Thus have I instructed you on Samādhi which leads to Liberation. Rāja-yoga-samādhi, Unmanī, Sahajāvasthā, they all mean union with the Self (Ātman)."

If the end of the Vedas is, truly, not Vedānta but Yoga, the end of Yoga is Samādhi.

A few more quotations from several scriptures may be welcome here, and the reader may find it useful to take to heart some of the hints given in them as later he comes to study the Pure Yoga of the Gheraṇḍa-saṃhitā in the light of our commentary, which should prove, we hope, as a kind of Ariadne's thread leading the intelligent and honest seeker after truth, through the maze of this sublime Yoga, to the very Heart of Reality.

It is said in the Triśikhī-brāhmaṇa Upaniṣad:

> वित्तस्य निश्चलीभावो धारणा धारणं विदुः।
> सोऽहं चिन्मात्रमेवेति चिन्तनं ध्यानमुच्यते।
> ध्यानस्य विस्मृतिः सम्यक् समाधिरभिधीयते। (31-32)

> "To hold the mind still is known as concentration.
> The pure, exclusive thought 'I am He', Pure Consciousness, is called contemplation.
> When the very thought of contemplation subsides, this is known as absorption (Samādhi)."

The Brahma-bindu Upaniṣad, in describing the process of meditation declares:

तावदेव निरोद्धव्यं यावत् हृदि गतं क्षयम् ।
एतत् ज्ञानं च मोक्षश्च अतोऽन्यो ग्रन्थविस्तरः ॥
निरस्तविषयासङ्गं सन्निरुद्धं मनो हृदि ।
यदा यात्युन्मनीभावं तदा तत् परमं पदम् ॥

"The mind has to be controlled until it gets absorbed in itself. This absorption of the mind in itself is what is called Jñāna and Mokṣa. Saying more would be unnecessary elaboration.
When the mind, perfectly controlled, with no worldly attachment, gets absorbed, there arises the Supreme state of Liberation."

And, as if pin-pointing the process, the Tejo-bindu Upaniṣad states:

भ्रुवोर्मध्ये ललाटे तु नासिकायास्तु मूलतः ।
जानीयादमृतं स्थानं तत् ब्रह्मायतनं महत् ॥

"At the middle of the eye-brows, in the forehead and at the root of the nose is to be known the seat of nectar. That is the supreme abode of Brahman."

In time, as Rāja-yoga develops, all effort ceases, for, as rightly declared in the Garuḍa Purāṇa:

सम्प्राप्तयोगसिद्धिस्तु पूर्णो यस्त्वात्मदर्शनात् ।
न किञ्चित् दृश्यते कार्यं तेनैव सकलं कृतम् ॥

"He who has attained the Supreme Power of Yoga (Yoga-siddhi) through the visualization of the Ātman, becomes perfect. There is nothing else for him to do. He has discharged all his duties."

There is then neither a controller nor a controlled, neither a knower nor a known. As wisely put by Śaṅkarācārya in his Yoga-tārāvalī:

न दृष्टिलक्ष्याणि न चित्तबन्धो
न देशकालौ न च वायुरोधः ।
न धारणाध्यानपरिश्रमो वा
समेधमाने सति राजयोगे ॥

"As Rāja-Yoga develops, the eye need not be fixed on any goal, the mind need not be controlled; there are neither restrictions of time and place, nor the breath need be subdued, nor any effort be made to achieve Dhāraṇā and Dhyāna."

Such a true yogin can verily say, together with Śaṅkarācārya in his Hastāmalaka-stotra:

नाहं मनुष्यो न च देवयक्षौ
न ब्राह्मणक्षत्रियवैश्यशूद्राः ।
न ब्रह्मचारी न गृही वनस्थो
भिक्षुर्न चाहं निजबोधरूपः ॥

"I am neither man, nor god, nor Yakṣa. Neither am I Brāhmaṇa, Kṣatriya, Vaiśya or Śūdra. I am neither a celibate, nor a householder, neither a hermit nor a sannyāsin. I am truly the Form of the knowledge of Self or Jñānaśakti."

Such a yogin verily seeth all things in the Self and the Self in all things. He is the greatest among devotees. Of him, it can be rightly said, in the words of Śrīmad-bhāgavata:

सर्वभूतेषु यः पश्येद्भगवद्भावमात्मनः ।
भूतानि भगवत्यात्मन्येष भागवतोत्तमः ॥

"He who with his entire being perceives Divinity in all things and all things in Divinity, is the highest devotee."

To lead to THAT, is the whole purpose of the teachings of Gheraṇḍa-saṃhitā. To facilitate that, is the sole intention of this new work on Pure Yoga. He who reads otherwise, hasn't quite understood. He who thinks otherwise, is lacking in discrimination. Light to all. Peace to all.

OM... OM... OM...

Yogī Praṇavānanda

The First Lesson

ON THE YOGA OF THE PHYSICAL BODY

I BOW IN REVERENCE to that Ādi-īśvara who revealed the Science of Haṭha-yoga. It stands out as a ladder for those who aspire to reach the sublime heights of Rāja-yoga.

The term Ādi-īśvara means Supreme Lord or Ruler of our system of manifestation, of our world. It also means Supreme embodiment of Divine Consciousness, Love and Wisdom. According to Patañjali, "Īśvara is a particular Puruṣa who is untouched by the afflictions of life, actions and the results and impressions produced by these actions. In Him is the highest limit of Omniscience. Being unconditioned by time, He is Teacher even of the Ancients. His designator is OM."[4] Īśvara is the presiding Deity of this Solar System, Supreme Teacher (Guru) of all mankind for as long as this remains confined within this particular system. In Him 'we live and move and have our being'. In Śaṅkarācārya's view, "equalminded gurus teach, as the Vedas do, that the learned will be saved only by Wisdom derived from Īśvara (The Logos)".[5] This concept of the Logos (Word) permeates the various religious traditions existent in the world. It is found in Christianity, for example, in that gnostic passage of the Gospel according to St. John: "In the beginning was the Word, and the Word was with God, and the Word was God. The same was in the beginning with God. All things were made by Him; and without Him was not anything made that was made. In Him was life and the life was the light of men. And the light shineth in darkness, and the darkness comprehendeth it not."[6]

This Universe is not the result of a fortuitous concatenation of atoms and subatomic particles but the master product of the Logos, whose divine energy subtly directs and guides the whole process with infinite wisdom. To put it in the context of Yoga philosophy, "The tremendous effort and energy which is required in the manifestation of a universe comes from the Divine Will of Śiva, the Universal Consciousness, and appears, initially, through Ākāśa as Nāda or integrated 'Sound' from which all forms of vibration and modes of motion in the realm of manifestation are derived."[7] The path of Haṭha-yoga, when properly understood, represents a subtle 'mode of motion', and as such, it is rooted in that same Nāda or integrated 'Sound', the Word. This physical body itself is the product of that Holy Vibration.

ON THE YOGA OF THE PHYSICAL BODY

1. Once Caṇḍa-kāpāli went to Gheraṇḍa's hermitage, saluted him with reverence and devotion and asked of him—
Caṇḍa-kāpāli said:
2. O Greatest among the yogins! O Master of Yoga! O Lord! Instruct me now on the Yoga of the Physical Body which leads to the knowledge of Truth (Tattva-jñāna).
Gheraṇḍa replied:
3. Well asked, indeed, O mighty armed! I shall instruct you on what you ask. Attend to it with diligence.
4. There are no shackles like those of Illusion (Māyā), no power like that of Yoga, no better friend than Wisdom (Jñāna) and no greater enemy than Egoism (Ahaṃkāra).
5. As by learning the alphabet one can study all the sciences, so by thoroughly mastering this Yoga, one attains to Wisdom (Tattva-jñāna).
6. The bodies of all living beings are the result of good and bad deeds; the bodies give rise to actions (Karma) which lead to rebirth; the process continues like a rotating mill.
7. As the buckets in a rotating mill go up and down moved by the bullocks, now full, now empty of water, so the soul passes through life and death moved by its actions.
8. Like unto an unbaked earthen pot placed in water, the body soon decays (in this world). Bake it hard in the fire of Yoga in order to strengthen and purify it.
9. This Yoga is sevenfold: Purification, Strengthening, Steadying, Calming, Lightness, Perception and Isolation (Liberation).

'Instruct me now...', these words clearly indicate the nature of the relationship between guru and disciple and the stage of the latter on the path of Yoga. Caṇḍa-kāpāli is no newcomer, but rather an accepted disciple who has fulfilled certain preliminary requirements and who is in possession of certain qualifications and moral characteristics which make him fit and ready to tackle the problem of spiritual unfoldment in an intensive and serious manner; indeed, he is no newcomer but a worthy disciple in whom qualities of non-attachment and spiritual discernment are progressively coming into full bloom. These preliminary qualifications for discipleship have been described in theosophical literature with extreme lucidity in the following passage:

> "Behold the Truth before you: A clean life, an open mind, a pure heart, an eager intellect, an unveiled spiritual perception, a brotherliness for one's co-disciple, a readiness to give and receive advice and instruction, a loyal sense of duty to the Teacher, a willing obedience to the behests of Truth, once we have placed our confidence in, and believe that Teacher to be in possession of it; a courageous endurance of personal injustice, a brave declaration of principles, a valiant defence of those who are unjustly attacked, and a constant eye to the ideal of human progression and perfection, which the Secret Science (Gupta-vidyā) depicts; these are the Golden Stairs up the steps of which the learner may climb to the Temple of Divine Wisdom."[8]

The true nature of Haṭha-yoga (the Yoga of the physical body) has been very much misunderstood both in the West and in the East. Therefore, it is somewhat refreshing to read in one of Dr. Taimni's excellent books on Yoga the following: "Haṭha-yoga concentrates on the form and by the proper scientific manipulation of forces working in our vehicles aims to bring about changes in consciousness. But this method is meant only for very advanced souls who have already conquered their desires and lower nature and who have only to establish operational relationships between the lower and higher vehicles. Rāja-yoga on the other hand concentrates on the unfoldment of consciousness and lets the vehicles adjust themselves slowly and naturally to the changes in consciousness."[9] Yes, Haṭha-yoga concentrates on the form, but its movement is from the form to the formless, from the form to the consciousness that ensouls it. That true Haṭha-Yoga does not neglect consciousness will become clearer as the reader proceeds, for there is more to this Yoga than meets the ordinary eye.

Before a soul can realize its full potential it must perforce pass through life and death not once but many, many times, moved by its actions. Gheraṇḍa compares this process to a rotating mill. It is the process of reincarnation (the wheel of births and deaths). A clear trace of this idea or doctrine is present also in the Christian Gospels most definitely in at least three different places, as indicated by the verses that follow:

> "And if you will receive it, this is Elias, which was for to come.
> He that hath ears to hear, let him hear."[10]

and,

> "And his disciples asked him saying, Master, who did sin, this man or his parents, that he was born blind?"[11]

and,

> "Him that overcometh will I make a pillar in the temple of my God, and he shall go no more out..."[12]

'Him that overcometh' being none other than man made perfect: a Master of Yoga.

10-11. Purification is achieved by the regular performance of six practices (Ṣaṭkarma-s): Āsanas or postures give Strength (Dṛḍhatā); Mudrās give Steadiness (Sthiratā); Pratyāhāra gives Calmness (Dhīratā); Prāṇāyāma gives Lightness (Laghiman); Dhyāna gives Perception of Self (Pratyakṣatva) and Samādhi confers Independence (Nirliptatā) which is verily Liberation. MOKSHA

12. (A) Dhauti, (B) Vasti, (C) Neti, (D) Laulikī, (E) Trāṭaka and (F) Kapālabhāti are the Ṣaṭkarma-s or six purificatory practices, known as Sādhana.

(A) The four internal Dhautis

13. The Dhautis are of four kinds; they clear away the impurities of the body. They are: (a) Antar-dhauti (internal cleansing), (b) Dantadhauti (cleaning the teeth), (c) Hṛd-dhauti (cleaning the heart) and (d) Mūlaśodhana (cleaning the rectum).

(a) ANTAR-DHAUTI

14. Antar-dhauti is again subdivided into four parts: Vātasāra (air purification), Vārisāra (water purification), Vahnī-(or

Agni) sāra (fire purification) and Bahiṣkṛta (external purification).

VĀTASĀRA-DHAUTI

15. With mouth contracted like the beak of a crow, drink air slowly, filling the stomach; then move it therein, and slowly expel it through the lower passage.
16. The Vātasāra should be kept very secret. It causes purification of the body; destroys all diseases and increases the gastric fire.

It has been said that ninety per cent of the ills that afflict human beings have their origin in an impure digestive system. The alimentary canal, beginning with the oesophagus and ending with the rectum is some twenty-seven feet in length, and although nature periodically cleanses it, this yoga practice is intended to ensure that the cleansing is complete. By passing a current of air through the tortuous tract, oxidation of the foetid products, noxious and deleterious gases, etc. is produced. The digestive surface of the alimentary canal is extraordinarily vast and complex; their cells are experts at allowing foodstuff, when properly disgested, to penetrate the body and to nourish it, whilst bacteria and other harmful products are normally held in control by the intestinal membrane and the defence mechanism protecting it. Vātasāra ensures a healthy membrane; it tones and revitalises the entire system. It is obvious that the personal and delicate nature of such hygienic practice makes it imperative that one keeps it to oneself; therefore, 'it should be kept very secret'.

VĀRISĀRA-DHAUTI

17. Fill the gullet with water and then drink it slowly; then, move it through the stomach, forcing it outwards through the rectum.
18. The Vārisāra is to be kept very secret. It purifies the body. By practising it with ease and care, one gets a body radiantly healthy.
19. The Vārisāra is the best of all Dhautis. He who diligently practises it, purifies his impure body and turns it into a shining one.

A more effective and perhaps even pleasant way of cleansing the intestinal tract is by means of this Vārisāra-dhauti. It consists in drinking various glasses of salty water (to such I would add a couple of spoonfuls of fresh lemon juice). Then, by performing Uḍḍīyāna-bandha (see Third Lesson, 10-11) the water passes mechanically into the long intestine. Finally, by means of Laulikī (see verse 52) the water passes into the large intestine and in a matter of minutes is expelled through the rectum. The complete success of this practice depends on the correct performance of Uḍḍīyāna-bandha and Laulikī, which, in turn, may take a few months to master. This practice is totally harmless and, according to the text, 'the best of all Dhautis'.

AGNISĀRA-DHAUTI

20. Press in the navel knot towards the spine one hundred times. This is the Agnisāra or fire process which gives success in the practice of Yoga. It cures all stomach diseases and increases the internal (gastric) fire.
21. This Dhauti should be kept very secret; it is difficult to attain even by the gods. By this practice alone one verily gets a radiant body.

This practice increases the gastric fire, prevents dyspepsia, gastroenteritis, constipation, acidity and all sort of stomach diseases. Pancreas and liver improve their performance as a result of the intestinal massage. There is considerable increase of the appetite and unnecessary—often unsightly—fat deposits are progressively reduced. The body becomes firm and luminous. The figure 'one hundred times' should be reached very gradually, without excessive effort; starting with—say—ten to twelve times and increasing weekly.

BAHIṢKṚTA-DHAUTI

22. By means of Kākī-mudrā or crow-beak mudrā, fill the stomach with air, hold it there for one hour and a half and then force it towards the intestines. This practice should be kept very secret. It must not be divulged.
23. Then, standing in navel-deep water, draw out the Śaktināḍī

(long intestines), wash the Nāḍī with the hands, until it is perfectly clean; with care, it should then be drawn in into the abdomen.

24. This practice should be kept secret. It is not easily attained even by the gods. By means of this practice one gets Deva-deha (Godlike body).
25. This great Dhauti cannot be achieved for as long as a person has not gained the power of retaining air in the stomach for an hour and a half.

This rather formidable practice consists of the partial removal of the large intestines from the body, thoroughly cleaning them (washing them out) and replacing them in the original position. It is a risky practice which only a proficient master can accomplish and should never be undertaken without competent guidance. It may well lead to prolapsus and other serious complications. Moreover, he who has mastered the previous practices will find this extreme Dhauti unnecessary and superfluous. It does indicate, however, the meticulous thoroughness of the yogic approach and the yogin's competence in practical physiology.

He who would practise this internal cleansing (Dhautis) should always proceed from the 'gross' to the 'subtle', from the more material to the less material; the natural progression here being Uḍḍīyāna, Laulikī, Vārisāra, Vātasāra and Agnisāra; or, Earth, Water, Air and Fire. This movement from the 'gross' to the 'subtle' is always one of the keys to the proper understanding of Yoga.

(b) DANTA-DHAUTI

26. Five practices constitute Danta-dhauti : washing of the root of teeth [gums] {Danta-mūla-dhauti}, of the tongue (Jihvā-śodhana)" of the ear openings (Karṇa-Dhauti) and of the frontal sinuses (Kapāla-randhra-dhauti).

DANTA-MŪLA-DHAUTI

27. Rub the teeth (gums) with catechu-powder or with pure earth until all dental impurities are removed.
28. This washing of the teeth (gums) is a great Dhauti among

yogins. It should be done every morning in order to preserve one's teeth. The yogins highly recommend this purificatory practice.

The really important thing is the intelligent and persistent massaging of the gums and not so much the brushing of the teeth so greatly popularised in the West, which in fact often produces the opposite effect.

JIHVĀ-ŚODHANA-DHAUTI

29. I shall now explain to you the method of cleansing the tongue. The elongation of the tongue destroys disease, old age and death.
30. Join together the three fingers known as the index, the middle and the ring finger, placed them into the throat in the right manner and, slowly, rub well the root of the tongue and by washing it, expel the phlegm.
31. Rub the tongue with butter, and milk, repeatedly. Then, by carefully holding the tip of the tongue with an iron instrument, pull it out gradually and slowly.
32. Be this your daily practice before the rising and setting of the sun. By so doing, the tongue becomes elongated.

The rubbing (scraping) of the root of the tongue prevents the accumulation of phlegm which occurs throughout the years, and which is responsible for stale breath and general lack of freshness in one's mouth; it keeps at bay throat infections, even tooth decay. The manipulation (milking) of the tongue stimulates the inner recesses of the oral cavity and greatly adds to the perfect functioning of the various glands in the deep of the neck, i.e. thyroid, parathyroids and thymus. It constitutes excellent preparation for the more advanced Yoga practices. The scraping should be done gently and not too deeply in order to prevent possible nausea.

KARṆA-DHAUTI

33. Rub the two ear-holes with the index and ring finger. By such daily practice the mystical sounds (Nāda) are heard.

One should not take the results achieved by this simple practice too literally, for what is indicated here is much more than a simple rubbing of one's ears. It indicates a deep state of concentration on the faculty of hearing whereby, eventually, some mystical sounds (Nāda) are heard. These sounds ought not to be confused with the cardio-vascular noises also audible to the Yogin. This practice tends to induce sharpness of hearing, and later-much later (when other conditions of higher Yoga are fulfilled)—clairaudience.

KAPĀLA-RANDHRA-DHAUTI

34. Rub with the thumb of the right hand the depression in the forehead, by the root of the nose. Such practice cures all phlegmatic disorders.
35. The Nāḍīs become purified and clairvoyance is induced. This should be practised daily on awakening from sleep, after meals and in the evening.

Not only does this practice improve physical sight but, bearing in mind what has just been said about the previous Dhauti, it also, eventually, induces clairvoyance.

(c) HṚD-DHAUTI

36. The purification of the heart (or rather the throat) is threefold: by a stick (Daṇḍa), by vomiting (Vamana) and by a piece of cloth (Vāsas).

DAṆḌA-DHAUTI

37. Thrust either a plantain stalk or a stalk of turmeric (Haridrā) or a stalk of cane slowly into the gullet and then draw it out also slowly.
38. This practice will expel all the phlegm, bile and other impurities out of the mouth. By this Dhauti all heart diseases are surely cured.

VAMANA-DHAUTI

39. After meals, the intelligent practitioner should drink water enough to fill the stomach up to the throat, then, after hav-

ing looked for a while upwards, he should vomit it out. This daily practice cures all disorders of the phlegm and bile.

VĀSO-DHAUTI

40. Swallow slowly a thin cloth, four fingers wide, then draw it out again. This is called Vāso-dhauti.

41. This practice cures Gulma (chronic gastritis), fever, enlarged spleen, leprosy, and other skin diseases and disorders of phlegm and bile; and the practitioner finds his health, strength and cheerfulness increasing day by day.
Hṛd-dhauti is threefold and is somewhat analogous to 'washing the dishes' thoroughly, i.e. with a stalk, with water and with a cloth. The latter practice requires a certain amount of skill and patience. The cloth should be very fine and seamless (about 15 feet long and 3 inches wide) perfectly clean and soaked in warm water. One should learn to swallow it slowly at first (not in a lump) a little bit at a time (about a foot) increasing it gradually until one can swallow the whole length without discomfort in one attempt. The cloth should be kept in the stomach for about 5 minutes, then, it should be carefully withdrawn. The operation is greatly facilitated by drinking some warm water just before proceeding to withdraw the cloth from the stomach.

(d) MŪLA-ŚODHANA

42. The Apāna-vāyu (wind, gas) does not flow freely so long as the rectum is not purified. Therefore, one must take the greatest care in practising the purification of the large intestines.

43. By the stalk of the root of Haridrā (turmeric) or the middle finger, one should cleanse the rectum carefully with water.

44. Such practice destroys constipation, indigestion and dyspepsia; it increases the beauty and vitality of the body and kindles the gastric fire.

(B) VASTIS

45. There are two kinds of Vastis described: Jala-vasti (or water Vasti) and Śuṣka-vasti (or dry Vasti). Water Vasti is always done in water, and dry Vasti always on land.

JALA-VASTI

46. Entering water up to the navel and adopting the posture Utkaṭāsana, one should contract and expand the sphincter muscle of the anus, repeatedly. This is called Jala-vasti.
47. This cures Prameha (urinary disorders), Udāvarta (digestive disorders) and Krūravāyu (flatulence, wind disorders). One's body becomes free from all diseases and as beautiful as that of the god Cupid.

ŚUṢKA-VASTI

48. Adopting the posture called Paścimottāna, move the intestines slowly downwards, then contract and expand the sphincter-muscle of the anus with Aśvinī-mudrā.
49. This practice prevents constipation and it increases the gastric fire and cures flatulence.
Jala-vasti is the equivalent to the western enema (that old remedy so much in neglect nowadays) except that it is not an entirely mechanical thing. It requires the control of the sphincter-muscle of the anus and the mastery of Uḍḍiyāna-bandha (see Third Lesson, 10-11) and Laulikī (see verse 52). It also stimulates the bladder. That is why it is claimed to cure all urinary disorders.

Śuṣka-vasti is purely muscular (dry); it combines the Paścimottāna posture (see Second Lesson, 26) with Aśvinī-mudrā (see Third Lesson, 82-83) and it tones the abdominal organs and keeps them free from sluggishness. It also stimulates the kidneys and spine and constitutes excellent preparation for the more advanced Yoga practices.

(C) NETI

50. Pass a thin thread measuring about 10 inches right through

the nostrils and pull it out by the mouth. This is called Neti-kriyā.

51. By this practice, one obtains Khecarī-siddhi. It eliminates the disorders of phlegm and produces clairvoyance and clear sight.

One could safely use a fine catheter instead of a thread. As for the reference to obtaining Khecarī-siddhi, one should not take this too literally and what has been said earlier in connection with verses 33 and 35 also applies here. For a clearer understanding of the meaning of this verse one should refer to the lesson on Mudrās.

(D) LAULIKĪ

52. Forcefully move the abdominal contents from one side to the other. This is called Laulikī-yoga. It destroys all diseases and increases the gastric fire.

This practice consists of the isolation and rolling of the 'rectus abdominis', the straight muscles of the abdomen. Only he who has mastered Uḍḍīyāna is ready to attempt this practice. Adopting the semi-squatting position, the hands should rest on the thighs with fingers pointing inwards. The rolling motion should take place from right to left and vice-versa. Needless to say, one requires to be able to control the breath to a certain extent, and the practice should be done only on an empty stomach.

(E) TRĀṬAKA

53. Without winking, gaze steadily at any small object until tears begin to flow. The wise call this practice Trāṭaka.

54. Success in this practice leads to Śāmbhavī-mudrā. It cures all diseases of the eyes and induces clairvoyance.

Problems of myopia (shortsightedness) and presbyopia (longsightedness) can be very much improved, avoided and, in some cases even eliminated altogether by the regular and correct performance of this practice; especially if one chooses various objects at various distances and learns to combine the 'wandering' with the 'rigid' gaze. Such practice tones the whole nervous system. If improperly carried out, however, it may induce hypnosis and even produce serious disorders.

There are various types of Trāṭaka, i.e. (1) with eyes fixed on the tip of the nose, (2) with eyes fixed between the two eyebrows, (3) right shoulder gaze, (4) left shoulder gaze, and (5) on various objects such as a flame, a light, water, the sun, the moon, etc. Finally, Trāṭaka on 'mid-air'. He who knows this last practice becomes a knower of Śāmbhavī-mudrā, without a doubt. There exists a subtle but direct relationship between the gaze and the centre of command (Ājñā-cakra). Proficiency in true Trāṭaka leads to Śāmbhavī-mudrā, the sign of perfect concentration. By steadying the gaze, one's eyes become like those of a bird incubating an egg. The idea behind Trāṭaka being that if the gaze remains steady, then, the stream of thought also remains steady, continuous, uninterrupted. Trāṭaka aims to become Śāmbhavī-mudrā by a method of induction, so to speak. It is because in the beginning of all Yoga practices one comes to notice that the eyes of him who is absorbed remain naturally fixed, that the technique of Trāṭaka evolves into a Yoga technique. How useful it really is most surely depends on how wisely one uses it. Much of what at present passes for Rāja-yoga is based upon a misguided interpretation of this Trāṭaka and in the majority of cases it induces hypnotic sleep and can only lead to Jaḍa-(false) samādhi. "Converting the ordinary vision into one of knowledge one should view the world as Brahman Itself. That is the noblest vision, and not that which is directed to the tip of the nose."[13] (More on Śāmbhavī-mudrā in Third Lesson, 64, and Sixth Lesson, 20.)

(F) KAPĀLABHĀTI

55. The Kapālabhāti is threefold: Vāma-krama, Vyut-krama and Śit-krama. Through these, all disorders of the phlegm are destroyed.

VĀMA-KRAMA

56. Breathe in through the left nostril and out through the

right one; breathe in through the right nostril and out through the left one.

57. The inspiration and expiration must be effortless. All disorders of the phlegm are destroyed by this practice.

VYUT-KRAMA

58. Draw water through both nostrils and expel it through the mouth, very slowly. This is known as Vyut-krama, the destroyer of all phlegmatic disorders.

ŚIT-KRAMA

59. Suck water noisily through the mouth and expel it through the nostrils. By this Yoga practice one becomes like the god Cupid.

60. Neither old age nor fever ever touches him. Disorders due to phlegm are destroyed and the body becomes healthy and supple, obedient to his will.

The cleansing of the frontal cavity (frontal sinus) is done by Kapālabhāti, which can be 'dry' or 'wet'. The 'wet' practices should be carried out carefully, always making sure that one has sufficient air in the lungs to cope with any unexpected emergency, i.e. in case some of the water finds its way into the air passages, so that it may be easily expelled. The water should be warm with a little lemon juice in it, to increase the prophylactic side of such practices. Colds, catarrhs, hay fever, headaches, sore throats, are cured or held at bay without a doubt. The 'dry' practice serves as preparation for the exercises of Prāṇāyāma—apart from inherent therapeutic virtues. It purifies the Nāḍīs (subtle channels of cosmic energy—Prāṇa) and establishes a gentle rhythm throughout the whole organism.

All the foregoing practices, according to this particular Yoga treatise, constitute the stage of 'Purification'. Any serious practitioner soon discovers that, although the expressions 'radiant body', 'death destroyer', 'God-like body' and so on may appear somewhat exaggerated, the principles inspiring them are highly scientific and reasonable, and, from the therapeutic and prophylactic point of view, highly effective. The body soon decays—this is an unavoidable fact of life. The Yogin aims at converting his body into a Diamond Body, a suitable instrument for the unfoldment of his higher possibilities. Purity leads to strength. On such a sound foundation the Yogin can build to his heart's content. Time is a very important factor in the process of Liberation from the point of view of Yoga; a sound, healthy, efficient and long lasting body provides not only excellent material conditions for the Yogin, but time in which to unfold, time in which to transform himself, time in which to attempt to reach the other shore, time in which to master Yoga.

The Second Lesson

"Āsanas make one firm, free from
maladies and light of limb."

(Haṭha-yoga-pradīpikā, I, 17)

"One should know that to be real
posture in which the meditation
of Brahman flows spontaneously
and unceasingly, and not any
other that destroys one's happiness."

(Aparokṣānubhūti of Śrī-saṅkarācārya, verse 112)

ĀSANAS

Gheraṇḍa said:

1. There are as many Āsanas (postures) as there are numbers of species of living creatures in this universe. Of these, Śiva has described eighty-four hundreds of thousands.
2. Among them, eighty-four are the best, and among these eighty-four, thirty-two have been found useful for mankind in this world.
3. Siddha, Padma, Bhadra, Mukta, Vajra, Svastika and Siṃha, Gomukha, Vīra and Dhanur;
4. Mṛta, Gupta, Matsya, Matsyendra, Gorakṣa, Paścimottāna, Utkaṭa and Saṅkaṭa;
5. Mayūra, Kukkuṭa, Kūrma, Uttāna-kūrma, Uttāna-maṇḍuka, Vṛkṣa, Maṇḍuka, Garuḍa, Vṛṣa;
6. Śalabha, Makara, Uṣṭra, Bhujaṅga, and Yoga are the thirty-two Āsanas that give perfection (Siddhi) in this mortal world.

The word 'Siddhi' is variously translated as achievement, perfection, wisdom, accomplishment, psychic power, control, mastery, Kaivalya, Nirvāṇa and Self-Realization. It is important to bear in mind that the word, as here used, is indicative of all such meanings. The most succinct and at the same time most important guiding line with regard to Āsanas has been given by Patañjali in his Yoga-sūtras:

II, 46. Posture (should be) steady and comfortable.
II, 47. By relaxation of effort and meditation on the 'Endless' (Ananta) posture is mastered.

Needless to say, success in one's meditation on the 'Endless' is in itself a considerable achievement in Yoga and therefore an Āsana perfectly mastered is much more than a simple posture; it implies mastery over certain subtle processes as well. The benefits of the various Āsanas are physical, psychological, psychic and psycho-spiritual. The sphere of influence of an Āsana extends to the following systems: Circulatory, Lymphatic, Endocrine,

Nervous, Prāṇic and Suṣumnā. The natural progression being, once again, from the 'gross' to the 'subtle'. The Mudrā practice as described in the next lesson represents the crown of the Āsana.

Many are the specific benefits of the various Āsanas. It all depends, however, on the degree of perfection achieved, and on the areas of the 'body' which are being stimulated (harmonised, affected) by the various postures, i.e. Vajrāsana, if practised immediately after eating, improves and accelerates the digestion; it is also ideal for meditation, a favourite Āsana with certain monastic orders. Siṃhāsana strengthens the muscles and organs of the neck, eyes, chest and spine; it stimulates the salivary glands and ensures healthy tonsils; it also affects the Thymus gland. Vṛkṣāsana improves the flexibility of the spinal column so important to Yoga and leads to greater mastery of one's nervous system, stimulates all the organs in the pelvic region, confers emotional stability and confidence in oneself, induces balance and breathing improves considerably.

One could sing the virtues of the various Āsanas almost ad infinitum; such is the enormous potential enshrined in the human body. There are available in the market a great many good books on the subject with hundreds of visual illustrations. The true Yogin experiments, chooses and masters. In the end, one Āsana is all one needs. Padmāsana? Vajrāsana? Siddhāsana? Truly, when one of them is mastered, of what use are the various other Āsanas?

1. SIDDHĀSANA (Perfect posture)

7. Place one heel at the anal aperture and the other on the root of the genitals. Then, rest your chin upon the chest and remain still. With senses subdued, gaze at the spot between the two eye-brows. This is called Siddhāsana which opens the door to freedom.

Men should place the left heel at the anal aperture, the right against the pubic bone. Women should use the opposite heels, on account of the rule of magnetic polarity. The spine should be kept erect and consciously relaxed; the gaze fixed straight ahead, focused, so to speak, in mid-air, naturally relaxed and not turned in (as often translated) and fixed between the eye-brows or on the tip of the nose! The awareness (consciousness) should be fixed (directed) to the inner spot between the two eye-brows. The gaze is properly 'fixed' when it is perfectly relaxed and poised in the void. Squinting and other false Haṭha-yoga practices produce the opposite result to the one intended, apart from causing various eye troubles and neurophysiological disorders, if carried to extremes.

Many are the benefits of this particular Āsana. It considerably improves the blood circulation in the pelvic region and tonifies the gonads. It is ideal for balancing the various prāṇic currents which circulate throughout the body, and the establishment of harmony in the whole body-system. The Haṭha-yoga-pradīpikā, another well-known Yoga classic, highly praises and recommends this Āsana in the words: "Of the eighty-four postures, one should always practise Siddhāsana. It purifies the 72,000 Nāḍīs. The Yogin who, contemplating the Self and following a moderate diet, continually practises the Siddhāsana during twelve years, obtains fulfilment. When the Siddhāsana is mastered, of what use are the various other Āsanas?..."[14] The importance of this and some of the other Āsanas will become clear when we come to study the lesson on Mudrās. For elucidation on the expression 'which opens the door to freedom', for example, one should consult Mudrā 12 (Śakticālanī).

2. PADMĀSANA (Lotus posture)

8. Place the right foot on the left thigh and the left foot on the right thigh and crossing the hands behind the back, firmly catch hold of the great toes. Rest the chin on the chest and fix the gaze on the tip of the nose. This is called Padmāsana, the destroyer of all diseases.

3. BHADRĀSANA (Gentle posture)

9. Place both heels crosswise under the perineum, carefully. Cross the hands behind the back and catch hold of the big toes.
10. Having adopted the Mudrā called Jālandhara, fix the gaze on the tip of the nose. This is Bhadrāsana (happy posture) which heals all sorts of diseases.

4. MUKTĀSANA (Free posture)

11. Place the left heel at the root of the genitals and the right heel above that; keep head, neck and body straight. This Muktāsana confers Siddhi (perfection).

5. VAJRĀSANA (Diamond posture)

12. Tighten the thighs hard as diamond and place the feet by the two sides of the anus. This is called Vajrāsana that gives perfection (Siddhi) to the Yogin.

6. SVASTIKĀSANA (Prosperous posture)

13. With body straight, sit with both feet between the legs and thighs, firmly locked. This is known as Svastikāsana.

7. SIṂHĀSANA (Lion posture)

14. Place the two heels under the perineum (each on the opposite side) with soles turned upwards; hands to rest on the knees which should touch the ground.

15. Open your mouth as you perform the Jālandhara-mudrā (chin lock) and fix your gaze on the root of the nose. This is Siṃhāsana, the destroyer of all diseases.

8. GOMUKHĀSANA (Cow-mouth posture)

16. Place both feet on the ground with heels crossed under the buttocks. Sit straight and still, the mouth raised. This is called Gomukhāsana, resembling the mouth of a cow.

9. VĪRĀSANA (Hero posture)

17. Place one foot on the opposite thigh and turn the other foot backwards. This is Vīrāsana.

10. DHANURĀSANA (Bow posture)

18. Stretch both legs on the ground like a stick and catching hold of the toes with the hands make the body like a bow. This is called Dhanurāsana or bow posture.

11. MṚTĀSANA (Corpse posture)

19. Lying flat on one's back, like a corpse is called Mṛtāsana. This posture dispels fatigue and induces calmness of mind.

12. GUPTĀSANA (Hidden posture)

20. Hide the feet between the knees and thighs with anus resting on the feet. This is known as Guptāsana.

13. MATSYĀSANA (Fish posture)

21. Adopting the Padmāsana posture but without crossing the arms, lie on the back, holding the head by the two elbows. This is the Matsyāsana, destroyer of all diseases.

14. MATSYENDRĀSANA (King of the fish posture)

22. Keeping both abdominal region and back at ease, sitting perfectly relaxed, bend the left leg and place it over the right thigh.

23. Then, place on this the elbow of the right hand, and place the face on the palm of the same hand, with gaze fixed between the eye-brows. This is called Matsyendra posture.

15. GORAKṢĀSANA (Gorakṣa posture)

24. Place the two feet, turned upwards, between the knees and the thighs, in a hidden way, the heels being covered by the two hands outstretched, facing upwards.

25. Contract the throat and fix the gaze on the tip of the nose. This is called Gorakṣāsana that gives success to the Yogins.

16. PAŚCIMOTTĀNĀSANA (Back-stretcher posture)

26. Stretch both legs on the ground, stiff like a stick and place the forehead on the knees catching the toes with both hands. This is called Paścimottānāsana.

17. UTKAṬĀSANA (Hazardous posture)

27. Keep the toes firm on the ground and the heels raised in

the air. The anus should rest on the heels. This is called Utkaṭāsana.

18. SAṄKAṬĀSANA (Twister/Danger posture)

28. Placing the left foot on the ground, twist the right leg around the left and place the two hands on the knees. This is known as Saṅkaṭāsana.

19. MAYŪRĀSANA (Peacock posture)

29. Place the palms of both hands on the ground, rest the navel on the two elbows and balance the body upon the hands with legs raised in the air and crossed like Padmāsana. This is called Mayūrāsana.

30. It destroys the effects of food poisoning, increases the gastric fire, counteracts the effects of deadly poisons; it easily cures diseases like chronic gastritis and fever. Such are the merits of Mayūrāsana.

20. KUKKUṬĀSANA (Cock posture)

31. Sitting in Padmāsana, thrust down the hands between the thighs and knees and heave the body which should be supported on the elbows. This is the cock posture.

21. KŪRMĀSANA (Trotoise posture)

32. Place the heels, cross-like fashion, under the perineum with head, neck and body straight. This is the tortoise posture.

22. UTTĀNAKŪRMAKĀSANA (Straight tortoise posture)

33. Adcpting the cock posture, catch hold of the neck with both hands, and stand stretched like a tortoise. This is the Uttānakūrmakāsana.

23. MAṆḌUKĀSANA (Frog posture)

34. Place both feet towards the back, looking upwards, the big

toes touching each other and the knees forward. This is called Maṇḍukāsana.

24. UTTĀNAMAṆḌUKĀSANA (Straight frog posture)

35. Adopt the frog posture and holding the head by the elbows, stand up like a frog. This is called Uttānamaṇḍukāsana.

25. VṚKṢĀSANA (Tree posture)

36. Standing straight on the left leg, bend the right leg and place the right foot on the root of the left thigh. Stand thus like a tree on the ground. This is called Vṛkṣāsana.

26. GARUḌĀSANA (Eagle posture)

37. Press against the ground with both legs and thighs and steady the body with the two knees placing both hands on them. This is called the Garuḍa posture.

27. VṚṢĀSANA (Bull posture)

38. Rest the anus on the right heel and place the left leg crossing over in the opposite direction, touching the ground. This is the bull posture.

28. ŚALABHĀSANA (Locust posture)

39. Lie on the ground with face downwards and both hands under the chest touching the ground with palms and both legs raised in the air ten inches high. This is called locust posture.

29. MAKARĀSANA (Dolphin posture)

40. Lie on the ground with face downwards and chest touching the ground, both legs stretched and head encircled by both arms. This is known as Makarāsana, which increases the gastric fire.

30. UṢṬRĀSANA (Camel posture)

41. Lie on the ground with face downwards and bend both legs towards the back with the help of the hands; mouth and abdomen to be contracted forcibly. This is the camel posture.

31. BHUJAṄGĀSANA (Cobra posture)

42. Let the body, from navel to toes, touch the ground, the palms placed upon the ground, and raise gently the upper part of the body (from navel to head) like a snake.
43. This posture increases the gastric fire; it destroys all diseases and by constant practice leads to the awakening of Kuṇḍalinī (the Serpent-goddess).

32. YOGĀSANA

44. Place both feet on the knees—soles upwards—and the hands on the ground with palms turned upwards.
45. Inspire and fix the gaze on the tip of the nose. This is Yogāsana adopted by the Yogins during their Sādhana (Training).

Thus ends the description of the thirty-two Āsanas that give perfection (Siddhi) in this mortal world. The true nature and the performance of the Āsanas become fully revealed in the next lesson, the Mudrā being the inner side of the Āsana.

The Third Lesson

"Carefully following this teaching,
he who concentrates on the practice
of the Mudrās, obtains the capacity
to overcome death, along with the
siddhis such as aṇiman."

(Haṭha-yoga-pradīpikā, III, 130)

MUDRĀS

Gheraṇḍa said:

1. There are twenty-five Mudrās whereby the Yogins attain success. They are as follows:
Mahā-mudrā, Nabho-mudrā, Uḍḍīyāna, Jālandhara, Mūlabandha, Mahā-bandha, Mahā-vedha, Khecarī,
2. Viparītakaraṇī, Yoni, Vajrolī, Śakticālanī, Tāḍāgī, Māṇḍukī, Śāmbhavī, Pañcadhāraṇās,
3. Aśvinī, Pāśinī, Kākī, Mātaṅginī and Bhujaṅginī.
4. Maheśvara, in addressing his consort, praised the value of Mudrās with the following words: "O Devi! I have explained to you the Mudrās; their knowledge (mastery) leads to adeptship.
5. It should be carefully kept secret and should not be revealed indiscriminately. It gives happiness to the Yogins and is difficult to attain even by the Maruts (gods of the air)."

The word Mudrā means 'seal', also 'mystery', 'secret'. It is the natural, inner extension of the previous stage, the Āsana. Mudrā depends greatly on the mastery of the Breath (Prāṇa) and Mind control. The Mudrā is the inner side of the Āsana. Inner control leads to perfect emancipation from one's complex bodily system. The practice of the various Mudrās leads to the eventual awakening of the powerful Goddess of Wisdom (Kuṇḍalinī) which abides semi-latent within the deepest recesses of the Yogin's subtle anatomy. Mudrās confer, among other, the so-called eight siddhis; these are: Aṇiman, the power to assume a minute (infinitesimal) form; Mahiman, the ability to assume a virtually all extensive form; Gariman, the power to become heavy; Laghiman, the power to become extremely light; Prāpti, the power to reach the most distant objects; Prākāmya, the power to obtain what is desired; Īśatva, the power to transform anything at will; and Vaśitva, the power to rule, to control anything. These great powers (Mahā-siddhis) indicate a certain level of attainment, or fulfilment by the Yogin, in so far as this world of manifestation is concerned. If the Yogin is not careful, they can become powerful temptations along the path of Yoga. When properly understood and mastered, Mudrās represent the meeting point of all Yogic disciplines and bear the seal of Liberation. The Mudrās form part of an integral whole—a most complex Mudrā-system—and fit within each other, so to speak, in the most harmonious manner. It makes nonsense, therefore, to consider and practise them separately. They are all secret, for they all refer to extremely subtle inner processes. They most certainly indicate very subtle inner disciplines and experiences and have absolutely nothing to do with the so often recommended techniques such as 'swallowing of the tongue', 'concentration on the tip of the nose', 'holding the breath', 'reversing the sex-current', and so many other false Haṭha-yoga practices which have brought the Sacred Science into disrepute; which have, indeed, almost destroyed it.

1. MAHĀ-MUDRĀ (Great seal)

6. Press carefully the left heel against the anus; stretch the right leg and catch hold of the toes with both hands.
7. Contract the throat and fix the gaze in the centre between the eye-brows. The wise call this Mahā-mudrā.
8. The practice of Mahā-mudrā cures consumption, constipation, enlargement of the spleen, indigestion and fever—all diseases in fact.

This Mudrā, when properly performed, provides not only physical benefits of various kinds, but it also brings into balance Iḍā-Piṅgalā System (see Fifth Lesson on Prāṇāyāma). It should be practised not only on the left but on the right side also. Like all Mudrās, it is to be understood esoterically. The Mudrā becomes really effective only when its subtle aspect is tapped or mastered.

2. NABHO-MUDRĀ (Heaven seal)

9. Wherever a Yogin may find himself, whatever he may do, let him ever keep his tongue turned upwards and always restrain his breath. This is the Nabho-mudrā, the destroyer of diseases of the Yogins.

The correct position of the tongue (with the root—not the tip—against the soft palate) ensures the automatic and perfect control of the breathing mechanism by the diaphragm, the only natural way of ensuring an ongoing complete breath. With diaphragmatic control secured, in time mastery of the Breath becomes an easy thing, relatively speaking. In its more subtle aspect, this Mudrā symbolizes an attitude of constant aspiration to the highest, the flame (tongue) reaching up towards the heavenly vault. It also represents an intimation of the King of Mudrās, the Khecarī-mudrā, the precursor of true Samādhi.

3. UḌḌĪYĀNA-BANDHA (Flying up control)

10. Contract the abdomen equally above and below the navel towards the back. By such practice the Great Bird (Breath) is forced to fly upwards. This Uḍḍīyāna-bandha is the lion that slays the elephant of death.
11. Of all Bandhas, Uḍḍīyana is the best. Mukti (Liberation) is naturally attained by him who follows this practice.

The expression 'Great Bird' refers to the flight upwards of Prāṇa or Kuṇḍalinī-śakti along the subtle Suṣumnā mechanism 'situated' in the central tube of the spinal cord.

4. JĀLANDHARA-BANDHA (Nectar-supply control)

12. Contract the throat and rest the chin on the chest. By this Jālandhara-bandha the sixteen Ādhāras are sealed. This great Mudrā annihilates death.
13. Success in the practice of Jālandhara-bandha confers Siddhis on the Yogins. He who practises for six months becomes a Siddha (Adept) without doubt.

The term 'Ādhāras' (substratum, supporting basis) refers to certain vital centres, the geography of which, in terms of physical anatomy, being as follows: The toes, the ankles, the knees, the thighs, the perineum, the genitals, the navel, the heart, the neck, the throat, the tongue, the nose, the centre of the eyebrows, the forehead, the head and the Brahmarandhra or upper opening of the Suṣumnā-nāḍī in the skull. It goes without saying that one requires more than just to contract one's throat and rest the chin on the chest to reap the benefits of this Mudrā. It is the complete mastery of a 'vital centre', sometimes called middle cakra (Viśuddha) that is here meant, and nothing less.

5. MŪLA-BANDHA (Root control)

14. Then, press the heel of the left foot against the perineum and contract the rectum, carefully pressing the navel against the spine.
15. The right heel is carefully placed on the root of the genitals. This annihilator of decay is called Mūla-bandha.
16. He who aspires to cross the Ocean of Saṃsāra (Death and Re-birth), let him practise this Mudrā in a secluded place, in secret.
17. By such practice, truly is mastery of Prāṇa achieved. So should one practise this, silently, diligently and with care.

Like all Mudrās, this particular Bandha is of deep spiritual significance; hence we read: "That (Brahman) which is the root of all existence and on which the restraint of the mind is based is called the restraining root (Mūla-bandha) which should always be adopted since it is fit for Rāja-yogins."[15]

6. MAHĀ-BANDHA (Great control)

18. Close the anus by the heel of the left foot and press that heel with the right foot carefully.
19. Move the heel gently (to stimulate the muscles of the rectum) and slowly contract the perineum whilst restraining the breath by Jālandhara-bandha. This is called Mahā-bandha.
20. Mahā-bandha is the greatest Bandha; it annihilates decay and death. By virtue of this Bandha, a man fulfils all his desires.

This Mudrā is simply the combination of the two preceding ones, a further step in the mastery of the complex Mudrā-system. No doubt a very important one, hence the name Mahā-bandha or Great Control.

7. MAHĀ-VEDHA (Great awakening)

21. As the beauty, charm and youth of women are as nothing without men, so are Mūla-bandha and Mahā-bandha without Mahā-vedha.
22. Having adopted the Mahā-bandha posture, restrain the breath by Uḍḍāna-kumbhaka. This is called Mahā-vedha, the giver of success to the Yogins.
23. The Yogin who daily practises Mahā-bandha and Mūla-bandha together with Mahā-vedha is the best of Yoga practitioners.
24. There is for such a Yogin no fear of death or old age. This Vedha should be kept carefully secret by the best among Yogins.

The mastery of the Breath by Uḍḍāna-kumbhaka (Uḍḍīyāna-bandha) is the element required for the great awakening. The idea is to drive the Prāṇa (Vital element) into the lower opening of the Suṣumnā-nāḍī. The instruction 'restrain the breath' should not be taken too literally. For clear elucidation of true Kumbhaka, one should refer to the subsequent lessons.

8. KHECARĪ-MUDRĀ (Seal of the heavenly flight)

25. Cut the lower tendon of the tongue and move the tongue constantly; rub it with fresh butter and pull it out with an iron pair of tweezers.
26. By such steady practice, the tongue lengthens and when it reaches the space between the eye-brows, Khecarī is achieved.
27. Turn the tongue backwards and upwards so as to touch the palate; when it reaches the holes of the nostrils opening into the brain cavity, and the gaze is directed to the space between the eye-brows, Khecarī results.

The word 'Khe' being a derivative-locative of 'Kha', here means: heaven, sky, air, ākāśa; and 'carī' has the sense of 'to roam', 'to wander', 'to loiter', etc. Sometimes, the siddhi gained by this Mudrā is understood too literally and most commentators claim that it allows the Yogin to 'fly through the sky', like a sort of competent Peter Pan, to become one of the 'denizens of the air', when what Khecarī really means is the conquest of that subtle, inner space (by the Kuṇḍalinī Fire) the external counterpart of which is the cranial cavity (between Ājñā and Sahasrāra). In the words of the Haṭha-yoga-pradīpikā: "When the prāṇa which is in the left and right Nāḍīs flows through the middle (Suṣumnā) in that state, the Khecarī-mudrā becomes perfect . . ."[16]

Khecarī-mudrā makes it possible for the fully vitalized and regenerated consciousness to remain firmly concentrated on the Ājñā-cakra, master of the Void, in pursuit of the total mastery of Ākāśa. Of this subtle and complex element, Sarasvatī, eternal and fleeting, mother of the Vedas and inspirer of Yogins, is made to say in that Hindu classic of Vedānta literature, the Yoga-vāsiṣṭha:

> "Of the three kinds of Ākāśa, namely Cidākāśa (Spiritual Ākāśa) Cittākāśa (Mental Ākāśa) and Bhutākāśa (Elemental Ākāśa) Cittākāśa is that intermediate state in which the mind is when it flits from one object to another in the elemental Ākāśa of objects. When the hosts of saṅkalpas in us perish, then the light of Cit, which is quiescent and immaculate and manifests itself as the universe, will shine in us. If one becomes convinced of the unreality of visible objects, then, through that Jñāna, he will attain Cidākāśa at once. Mayest thou attain through my grace that Cidākāśa."[17]

He who has mastered Khecarī-mudrā soon becomes convinced of the unreality of the visible universe; such knowledge (Jñāna) opens the gates to the spiritual realms (Cidākāśa).

But, how do most commentators understand and interpret this sublime Khecarī-mudrā? Quite literally, by learning to swallow one's tongue until it finally reaches the inner cavity, the space between the eye-brows!

The cases of false Haṭha-yogins who, 'mastering Khecarī', have from time to time allowed themselves to be buried alive only to emerge sound and well after a certain period of time, is well documented. The famous case of Haridāsa springs to mind as a feat of extraordinary endurance. Once he succeeded to spend 40 days buried underground (without food, water or air) after which time he was found to be alive and well. Years later, however, repeating some similar feat, something must have gone wrong, for he did not survive the experiment. It is a matter of conjecture whether his body ever became 'Deva-like' (radiant) or whether he at last had become complete master of the Ākāśa. It seems most certain that he was met by death.

28. Such practice prevents fainting, hunger, thirst and fatigue. There comes neither disease, nor old age, nor death. The body becomes radiant (Deva-like).
29. The body can neither be burned by fire, nor dried up by air, nor wetted by water, nor bitten by snakes.
30. It becomes beautiful; Samādhi is easily achieved and the tongue through contact with the holes in the cranium obtains various juices (nectar).
31. With the daily production of the various juices, one experiences new and blissful sensations; first comes a saltish taste, then alkaline, then bitter and then astringent.
32. Then, one feels the taste of butter, then of ghee, then of milk, then of curds, then of whey, then of honey, then of grape juice and, finally, arises the taste of nectar.

Although it is perfectly true that concentration upon the sensory organs (in this case the organ of taste, the tongue) does produce certain experiences of the nature described in verses 31 and 32, the real esoteric interpretation points in the direction of something much more sublime and subtle; the references to the various flavours in increasing range of delicacy and sweetness indicate several definite stages in Blissful Samādhi—the highest reaches of Yoga—until the accomplished Yogin tastes the heavenly nectar itself. That is why the text claims 'Samādhi is easily achieved' by such steady practice.

9. VIPARĪTAKARAṆĪ-MUDRĀ (Reversal seal)

33. The Sun abides in the root of the navel; the Moon in the root of the palate. As the Sun consumes the nectar, man becomes subject to death.
34. Bring the Sun upwards and the Moon downwards. This is

Viparītakaraṇī (Reversal control) held secret in all the Tantras.

35. Place the head on the ground with hands clasped around it, raise the legs up and thus remain immobile. This is called 'Reversal control'.

36. Practise this Mudrā constantly and you will destroy old age and death. You will become an Adept in all the worlds and will not perish even at Pralaya (world dissolution).

This Mudrā is also known as Śīrṣāsana (Head stand). It is said to be held secret in all the Tantras because the process is an extremely subtle and mysterious one. It refers to a reversal of inner magnetic polarity. The word 'Moon' stands for the Pineal-Pituitary System where the 'nectar' is being constantly produced. The word 'Sun' refers to the Solar Plexus region, the root of the navel or abdominal brain (Maṇipūra-cakra). It is said that the 'Sun' is always consuming the 'nectar' which descends from the 'Moon'. This Mudrā, by means of the reversal of inner polarity, activates the Suṣumnā mechanism whereby Kuṇḍalinī-śakti (see verse 49, Śakticālanī) also known as the slumbering Serpent Goddess, now awakens fully and blazes a trail of Consciousness and Bliss in her ascent along the mysterious Suṣumnā passage, deeply embedded within the Rod of Meru, in search of her consort Parama-śiva, towards the nuptial chamber of the Thousand-petalled Lotus (Sahasrāra). A radiant, imperishable 'body' is the product of such a lofty union ('to be spiritually minded is life'). Hence the claim, 'you will not perish even at Pralaya.' The delicate nature of this process or transformation is made somewhat more explicit by the description of Yoni-mudrā that follows.

10. YONI-MUDRĀ (Womb seal)

37. Sitting in Siddhāsana, the wise one closes the ears with the thumbs, the eyes with the index fingers, the nostrils with the middle fingers and the mouth with the ring and little fingers.

38. He draws in the Prāṇa-vāyu by Kākī-mudrā and joins it with the Apāna-vāyu contemplating the six cakras in their order and repeating the mantra Huṃ Haṃsa.

39. After he has awakened the sleeping Serpent-Goddess Kuṇḍalinī, let him lead the Śakti and the Jīva to the radiant lotus.
40. United to Śakti, let him aspire to the highest union with Śiva and the Supreme Bliss.
41. Let him contemplate on the union of Śiva and Śakti in this world, and being himself full of Spiritual Bliss, let him realize: 'I am Brahman' (The Supreme).
42. This Yoni-mudrā is the greatest secret, difficult to be attained even by the Devas. He who gains perfection in this practice becomes established in Samādhi.
43. He who steadily practises this Mudrā is never polluted by killing a Brāhmaṇa, killing a foetus, drinking liquor or polluting the bed of the Preceptor (Guru).
44. All mortal and venial sins are completely destroyed by the practice of Yoni-mudrā. Therefore, practise it if you aspire to Liberation.

The description of this Yoni-mudrā succinctly represents what is sometimes called variously Laya-yoga, Cakra-bheda, Kuṇḍalinī-yoga, and clearly refers to the delicate conquest of the Cakras. By means of such Unio Mystica, the body becomes a worthy vehicle for the expression of that Cosmic Fire which purifies and liberates the consciousness of the Yogin in an apotheosis of light. He who is born of such holy union has become forever karmaless; he is truly born again; he is a new creature. Hence the apparently exaggerated and contradictory (ridiculous being perhaps a better word) statements made in verses 43 and 44.

11. VAJROLĪ-MUDRĀ (Adamantine seal)

45. Place both palms on the ground, raise the legs upwards, the head in the air. This awakens the Śakti and prolongs life. The wise call it Vajrolī.
46. This practice is the best of all practices. It gives Liberation to the Yogins. By such auspicious practice the Yogins attain to Siddhis.
47. Bindu-siddhi (retention of seed) is easily attained by virtue of this practice. On the attainment of such Siddhi, what else can he not attain in this world?

48. Though engrossed in various pleasures, if he practises this Mudrā, all Siddhis will come to him.

This would seem to be a variation (a preparation perhaps) of the Viparītakaraṇī described earlier. Its main objective also being to awaken the Śakti from her slumber. The concept of 'Bindu-siddhi' ought to be esoterically understood and not as it is often the case in sexual terms.

ŚAKTICĀLANĪ (Raising the Śakti)

49. The great Goddess Kuṇḍalinī, the energy of the Self (Ātma-śakti) slumbers in the Mūlādhāra in the form of a snake, coiled up three and a half times.
50. So long as she slumbers in the body, the Jīva (soul) is like an animal and Wisdom does not arise, though one may practise ten million Yogas.

The text makes it quite clear that before any true spiritual awakening there must be first awakening of the Great Goddess Kuṇḍalinī. The Christian tradition refers to such awakening as 'the descent of the Holy Ghost'. And, although the nature of the awakening may take different forms, the liberating spiritual energy must always be present along the path of Yoga. Kuṇḍalinī can move, according to Hindu tradition, in five different fashions: (a) like an ant, crawling almost imperceptibly, (b) like a frog, bouncing unexpectedly, (c) like a snake, hissing and following a serpentine motion, (d) like a bird, following a direct or erratic flight, and (e) like a monkey, now holding to one branch, then to another. All depending on the chosen path of the Kuṇḍalinī-śakti.

51. As by a key a door may be opened, so may one, by awakening the Kuṇḍalinī by Haṭha-yoga, unlock the door of Brahman.

The expression 'awakening the Kuṇḍalinī by Haṭha-yoga' refers to the intelligent merging of Ha (Positive, Sun, Apāna, Individual Soul) and Ṭha (Negative, Moon, Prāṇa, Śiva), or the merging of Ha (Śiva) and Ṭha (Śakti) for the mystic union registers at different levels. It should not be understood—as it is often the case—as Haṭha-(forceful) yoga, i.e. by means of 'swallowing the tongue', 'holding the breath', 'reversing the sex current', and so many other misguided practices, for, as wisely remarked in the Yoga-vāsiṣṭha, 'Does not Haṭhayoga generate dire pain?'[18] It is because the word 'Haṭha' (spelled as a single word) means, 'force, violence, obstinacy, blow, stroke, forced meditation, etc.', that this fine Yoga has degenerated into all sort of superstitious practices, totally spurious to the true nature of Haṭha-yoga.

The expression 'door of Brahman' refers here to Mūlādhāra the lowest Cakra.

52. Wearing a loin-cloth, let him practise Śakticālanī in a secret room.
53. The loin-cloth should be one yard long and four fingers (3 inches) wide, white, soft and of fine texture. It should be joined with the Kaṭi-sūtra (a string worn around the loins).
54. Smear the body with ashes and, sitted in Siddhāsana, draw the Prāṇa-vāyu with both nostrils, forcibly joining it with Apāṇa.
55. Contract the rectum slowly by Aśvinī-mudrā, till the Vāyu vigorously enters the Suṣumnā, and manifests its presence.
56. By restraining the breath (Vāyu) during Kumbhaka in such manner the serpent Kuṇḍalinī, feeling suffocated, awakes and flies upwards to the Brahmarandhra.
57. Without Śakticālanī, the Yoni-mudrā remains fruitless. One should practise Śakticālanī first, then Yoni-mudrā.

The expressions 'restraining the breath' and 'forcibly joining Prāṇa with Apāna', ought not to be taken literally. The true meaning will emerge only with the understanding of this whole treatise. The reference to the fact that Śakticālanī should always precede Yoni-mudrā (Laya-yoga) prompts two obvious questions: (1) If that is so, why hasn't the author placed this verse in its proper place, following a natural and logical sequence? Even a cursory look at the text on Mudrās must have revealed by now that the author seems to have chosen to present these Yoga teachings entirely at random (everything seems to have been 'thrown in together' rather carelessly). This is true of this whole Haṭha-yoga treatise, as shall be explained later. (2) Is this apparent (obvious) confusion accidental or intentional? It is impossible to give any definite answer to either of these questions. However, it may be reasonable to assume that the writer's intention might have been to protect the Sacred Science from profane and unworthy eyes. In so doing, he may have done, in fact, more harm than good. That there is a definite sequence, a kind of Ariadne's thread which safely leads in and out of the labyrinth of Haṭha-yoga, should become evident to the reader as his understanding of the Sacred Science steadily grows, especially if the reader is also a keen and wise practitioner of Haṭha-yoga.

58. O Caṇḍakāpāli! Thus have I explained to you the Śakti-cālanī. Keep it carefully hidden and practise it daily.
59. This secret Mudrā conquers old age and death. Therefore, all Yogins, desirous of perfection, should practise it.
60. The Yogin who practises this steadily has Adeptship within his grasp; he attains Vigraha-siddhi (the ability to adopt any chosen form) and all his diseases vanish.

13. TĀḌĀGĪ-MUDRĀ (Tank seal)

61. Shape your abdomen to look hollow just like a tank. This is Tāḍāgī-mudrā, the destroyer of old age and death.

14. MĀṆḌUKĪ-MUDRĀ (Frog seal)

62. Close the mouth and move the root of the tongue towards the palate and taste the nectar gradually. This is known as Māṇḍukī-mudrā.
63. He who steadily practises Māṇḍukī-mudrā knows no wrinkles, nor old age; he retains perpetual youth; his hair never grows gray.

This is a kind of preliminary to Khecarī-mudrā and ought—like all Mudrās—to be understood esoterically. In saying this, one is not trying to deny certain physical benefits undoubtedly derived from the exoteric practice of the exercise.

15. ŚĀMBHAVĪ-MUDRĀ (Śambhu's seal)

64. Fix the gaze between the eye-brows and behold the Self-existent. This is Śāmbhavī, held secret in all the Tantras.

Sometimes people make no significant distinction between this Mudrā and Trāṭaka (see First Lesson, 54). "Fix the gaze between the eye-brows and behold the Self-existent." Such simple technique! How can it ever be kept secret? It is written that "He who knows the Śāmbhavī, is Brahman." Can such result be achieved by a simple technique? What is the real Śāmbhavī-mudrā, so praise-worthy? He who is master of Śāmbhavī appears to look into space-devoid of winking-whilst seeing nought; the gaze appears fixed, suspended in mid-space, void, whilst consciousness beholds the Self-existent; the eyes half opened, directed outwards, the awareness firmly established 'simultaneously' in the Heart and Head (Mind) via the 'citta-vāhā-nāḍī', hence the word 'Śāmbhavī'. To try to grasp Śāmbhavī by its external signs is to attempt to put the ocean in an empty bottle. That is why it is said to be held secret in all the Tantras.

65. The Vedas, the Śāstras and the Purāṇas are like public women, but this Śāmbhavī should be protected as if it were a respectable maiden.
66. He who knows this Śāmbhavī is like the Ādinātha (Lord of the World); he is Nārāyaṇa, he is Brahmā, the Creator.
67. "Truly, truly, and again truly",—said Maheśvara, "he who knows the Śāmbhavī, is Brahman. No one else."

16. THE FIVE DHĀRAṆĀ-MUDRĀS (Concentration seals)

68. The Śāmbhavī-mudrā has been explained; hear now about the Five Dhāraṇās. By means of these, what can't be accomplished in this world?
69. By this human frame one can visit and revisit Svargaloka; one can move through the air as swiftly as the mind.

With one's consciousness firmly established on the Self-existent, the Puruṣa, the size of a thumb of the Upaniṣads, forever present in the human Heart, one is enabled to proceed safely to the mastery of the five Tattvas (elements, subtle forces of Nature). These are known as Pṛthivī (Earth), Ambhas or Ap (Water), Agni or Tejas (Fire), Vāyu (Air) and Ākāśa (Ether). Mastery is achieved by means of five meditations. In the words of the Śiva-sūtra,

> "By the withdrawal of consciousness from the nāḍīs or channels along which vital forces flow in a vehicle, is attained mastery over the bhūtas (elements) and the capacity to isolate and separate them from one another."[19]

17. PṚTHIVĪ-DHĀRAṆĀ-MUDRĀ (Earth seal)

70. The Pṛthivī-tattva is yellow, has the letter (bīja) Laṃ as its secret symbol or seed; its form is four-sided and Brahmā is its presiding deity. By means of Kumbhaka, fix the Prāṇa and the Citta there for a period of five ghaṭikās (two hours). By this concentration (Adhodhāraṇā) one achieves mastery of the element Earth. It produces steadiness.
71. He who steadily practises this Dhāraṇā, becomes the champion of Death. Adept-like, he walks the earth.

Success in this concentration confers mastery over the Mūlādhāra-cakra which rules the Earth Tattva, with the consequent acquisition of Siddhis such as Telekinesis and Levitation.

18. ĀMBHASĪ-DHĀRAṆĀ-MUDRĀ (Water seal)

72. The beautiful Water-tattva is white like the moon, or a conch, or the Kunda flower; its form is circular like the moon and has the letter (bīja) Vaṃ as its ambrosial seed. Viṣṇu presides. Practising Kumbhaka, fix the Prāṇa and the Citta for five ghaṭikās there.
This is Āmbhasī-dhāraṇā, the destroyer of all ills and sorrows.
73. The Āmbhasī is a great Mudrā and he who masters it, is an expert Yogin. He never meets death even in frightful deepest water.

74. This great Mudrā should be kept carefully concealed. By disclosing it, one loses all chances of success—verily I tell the truth.

All ills and sorrows can be directly attributed to the misdirection of the creative energy in man. Hence the reference to "the destroyer of all ills and sorrows". Success in this concentration confers mastery over the Svādhiṣṭhāna-cakra which rules the Water-tattva, the sphere of the emotions. Walking on the waters and other precious Siddhis become readily achieved.

19. ĀGNEYĪ-DHĀRAṆĀ-MUDRĀ (Fire seal)

75. The Fire-tattva is situated in the navel; flaming red like the Indra-gopa insect, its form is triangular; it has the letter (bīja) Raṃ as seed, and is presided by Rudra, the giver of success. The Prāṇa along with the Citta should be fixed there for a period of five ghaṭikās. This Fire-Dhāraṇā dispels the dreadful fear of death.

76. Should the practitioner be thrown into a blazing fire, this Mudrā would keep him alive, without fear of death.

Success in this concentration confers mastery over the Maṇipūra-cakra which rules the Fire-tattva. Walking on fire and other Siddhis becomes readily achieved. A vivid description of this kind of Siddhi is to be found in the Book of Daniel, III, 21-25, where we read, "...I see four men loose, walking in the midst of the fire, and they have no hurt; and the form of the fourth is like the Son of God."

20. VĀYAVĪ-DHĀRAṆĀ-MUDRĀ (Air seal)

77. The Air-tattva is black as unguent for the eyes. It is full of Sattva quality; the letter (bīja) Yaṃ is its seed and Īśvara its presiding deity. The Prāṇa along with the Citta should be fixed in this Tattva for five ghaṭikās. This is the Vāyavī-dhāraṇā which enables the practitioner to move through the Air.

78. This great Mudrā conquers old age and death. Its practitioner need not fear death from any aerial accidents. It enables one to travel through the air.

79. This Mudrā should not be taught to the unworthy or those devoid of devotion. By so doing, all chances of success are lost. O Caṇḍa! This is verily the truth.

Success in this concentration confers mastery over the Anāhata-cakra which rules the Air-tattva. Travel through the Air (Kha) is to be understood here not as levitation, telekinesis, etc., but as the complex process of dematerialization and rematerialization. Hence the reference to 'devotion to Īśvara', the presiding deity and ruler of this system of manifestation, as a vital prerequisite.

21. ĀKĀŚĪ-DHĀRAṆĀ (Ether seal)

80. The Ether-tattva has the colour of the purest sea-water. Its seed (bīja) letter is Haṃ; it is presided by Sadāśiva. Fix the Prāṇa along with the Citta there for five ghaṭikās. This Ether-dhāraṇā unlocks the gates of Liberation (Mokṣa).
81. He who knows this Dhāraṇā is the real Yogin. Neither old age nor death touches him; and he does not perish during Pralaya.

Success in this concentration confers mastery over the Viśuddha-cakra, which rules the Ether-tattva. Sooner or later, this entire world process, this universe, will come to an end. The Yogin who is permanently established in the Ether has 'unlocked the gates of Liberation'; he has become 'karmaless', for, as it is written in Light on the Path, that little classic of theosophical literature, "He who desires to be karmaless must look to the air for home; and after that to the ether."[20] The Yogin is now free, by the proper combination of the five cosmic elements, to master the world of phenomena. Hence the reference, 'He does not perish during Pralaya.' However, that this mastery of the elements is not the ultimate end of Yoga is made absolutely clear by the following passage from the Śiva-sūtra:

> "In these lower siddhis or accomplishments there is still obscuration by moha or delusion of mind, caused by attachment which prevents complete freedom or Liberation from the world of manifestation."[21]

22. AŚVINĪ-MUDRĀ (Seal of the horse rider)

82. Contract and expand the anal aperture repeatedly. This is the Aśvinī-mudrā, the awakener of (Kuṇḍalinī) Śakti.
83. This Aśvinī is a great Mudrā. It eliminates all diseases of the rectum; it gives strength and vitality and prevents premature death.

This Mudrā differs from Jala- and Śuṣka-vasti (I, 46-49) in the fact that here both the concentration and the Prāṇa are vitally present and involved in the process. The regenerative agent is the Mystic Fire (Kuṇḍalinī-śakti) and not water.

23. PĀŚINĪ-MUDRĀ (Seal of the bird-catcher)

84. Throw both legs over the neck towards the back, and keep them strongly together as if held by a noose. This is the Pāśinī-mudrā which awakens the Śakti.
85. This great Mudrā confers strength and success. It should be diligently practised by those practitioners who aspire to perfection.

This Mudrā resembles a certain posture, 'Halāsana' (the plough); the main difference being that both the Prāṇa and the Citta are vitally involved. Kuṇḍalinī is sometimes referred to as 'The Great Bird', hence the allusion to the bird-catcher. It constitutes an excellent preparation for the awakening of Kuṇḍalinī-śakti.

24. KĀKĪ-MUDRĀ (Crow's seal)

86. With the mouth in the shape of the beak of a crow, drink the air very slowly. This is Kākī-mudrā that conquers all diseases.
87. This great Mudrā is kept secret in all the Tantras. By it, one becomes free from diseases like a crow.

This Mudrā resembles Vātasāra-dhauti, destroyer of all diseases. What then is its secret? The secret consists in understanding this Mudrā esoterically. It refers not to the drinking of air, but to the absorption, accumulation and distribution of

Prāṇa throughout the whole organism. By its very nature, it must remain secret.

25. MĀTAṄGINĪ-MUDRĀ (Elephant seal)

88. Standing in neck-deep water, draw in the water through both nostrils and expel it by the mouth.
89. Then, draw in the water through the mouth and expel it through the nostrils. This should be done repeatedly. It is called Elephant-Mudrā, destroyer of old age and death.
90. This Mudrā should be practised attentively in a secluded place free from human witnesses. By so doing, one becomes strong like an elephant.
91. Wherever he may be, the Yogin enjoys thus continuous comfort and pleasure. Therefore, this Mudrā should be practised with great diligence.

This looks, in appearance, very similar to Vyut- and Śīt-krama, the purificatory practices by means of water described in the First Lesson (I, 58-60). It has, however, a more esoteric sense to be discovered by the arduous and intelligent practitioner.

26. BHUJAṄGINĪ-MUDRĀ (Serpent seal)

92. Extruding the mouth a little forward, drink the air with the gullet. This is the Serpent-Mudrā, destroyer of old age and death.
93. This Mudrā quickly cures all abdominal diseases, especially indigestion, dyspepsia, etc.

This Mudrā also resembles Vātasāra-dhauti, destroyer of all diseases. It shares its secret with its predecessor, the Kākī-mudrā, and together form a set of advanced and subtle purificatory practices. The overt references to physical benefits are obviously a blind.

ON THE BENEFITS OF MUDRĀS

94. O Caṇḍa! Thus have I explained to you the lesson on Mudrās. They are highly treasured by all Adepts and destroy old age and death.

95. This should not be revealed indiscriminately: not to an unworthy person, nor to one devoid of true devotion. It should be carefully kept secret. It is difficult to attain even by the Devas.
96. These Mudrās should be revealed only to a sincere, honest and peace-minded person who is devoted to his Guru and comes from a good family. They confer happiness and liberation.
97. These Mudrās destroy all kinds of diseases and increase the gastric fire of him who practises them diligently.
98. To him death never comes, nor old age nor the like; he need not fear fire, water or air.
99. Cough, asthma, enlargement of the spleen, leprosy and phlegm diseases of twenty sorts, are most surely destroyed by the practice of these Mudrās.
100. O Caṇḍa! What more shall I tell you? In short, nothing in this world compares to the Mudrās for granting immediate success.

The Mudrā-system, when properly understood, is intended to cover the whole Yoga range. It deals superbly with Mantra, Haṭha, Laya, Kuṇḍalinī, Kriyā, Nāda, Bhakti, and Rāja-yoga. Nothing is left out. To the pure—he who has eyes to see and ears to hear—it represents a perfect whole where its various parts (Mudrās) form a fluidic sequence of subtle experiences, constantly proceeding from the 'gross' to the 'subtle'. These Mudrās, thrown in together in apparently careless disorder, stand as symbols of different orders of experience, where something always represents something else. They, together, form an integral system of cosmic proportions (a mighty Symbol), where all its various elements fit in perfect harmony, serving to give expression to the true purpose and goal of Yoga. It is, therefore, a mistake to think that one may readily isolate certain parts (techniques) in order to suit oneself. In doing this, one destroys the Mudrās; in doing this, one destroys Yoga. Yoga has to be taken 'whole'. This is also most true of the Mudrā-system. This view becomes extremely justifiable and clear the moment we proceed to introduce some kind of order into the puzzling disarray of Mudrās as given in the text. In examining the

Mudrās in their proper sequential order, they suddenly become less secret.

First, "whatever he may do, the Yogin should keep his tongue (flame) turned upwards"; wherever he should happen to be, he should always practise (1) Nabho-mudrā. Apart from the undoubted physical benefits conferred by this Mudrā, the aim is, most of all, to constantly remember 'whence one has fallen'; it represents constant aspiration to the Highest, to the Divine. (2) Bhujaṅginī-mudrā, (3) Mātaṅginī-mudrā and (4) Kākī-mudrā, would seem to belong here and constitute advanced and subtle purificatory practices. (5) Pāśinī-mudrā serves not only as a magnificent Āsana, it also prepares the awakening of the Kuṇḍalinī-śakti. (6) Vajrolī (Handstand) and (7) Viparīta-karaṇī (Headstand) follow next, and, apart from the considerable physical benefits they confer, they also form a 'living and dynamic' symbol of the return home, a gathering of psycho-spiritual energies (Reversal seal) for the inner journey. (8) Tāḍāgī-mudrā, followed by (9) Mahā-mudrā, serve to activate the Suṣumnā mechanism, with the help of the two 'witnesses', Iḍā and Piṅgalā (see Lesson Five on Prāṇāyāma); they serve as preparation for (10) Aśvinī-mudrā, naturally followed by (11) Uḍḍīyāna-bandha, (12) Mūla-bandha, (13) Jālandhara-bandha, (14) Mahā-bandha and (15) Mahā-vedha, which, together, form a perfect interlocking system paving the way for the raising of the great Goddess Kuṇḍalinī (16) Śakticālanī. Then follows (17) Yoni-mudrā, for, "without Śakticālanī, the Yoni-mudrā (Womb seal) remains fruitless..." (III, 57). Success in Yoni-mudrā ('the greatest secret'—every Mudrā always is the greatest secret!) paves the way to perfect concentration and mastery of the subtle elements (Tattvas); united to Śakti, the Yogin now proceeds to the conquest of the five Dhāraṇā-mudrās, (18) Pārthivī, (19) Āmbhasī, (20) Āgneyī, (21) Vāyavī and (22) Ākāśī-mudrā. Figuratively speaking, the Yogin has travelled from Mūlādhāra (lowest cakra) to Viśuddha (middle cakra) and is about to enter the Royal Path, the path of Rāja-yoga, in pursuit of the mastery of Manas-tattva (Cittākāśa). (23) Māṇḍuki-mudrā, apart from 'interlocking' the upper (Pituitary-Pineal) system, symbolizes the presence of the steady flame (tongue) of Liberation (like a candlelight in a windless place). (24) Śāmbhavī-mudrā, so praiseworthy, is none other than concentration on the Ājñā-cakra; without winking, seeing nought, the Yogin contemplates the Self-effulgent, peacefully absorbed. (25) Khecarī-mudrā symbolizes the final stages of this Yoga, the union of Ha (Individual Soul) with Ṭha (Śiva); the self to the SELF united. From Ājñā to Sahasrāra, along the most secret path, the wandering flame blazes a blissful trail, bringing to fulfilment a perfect unio mystica in the realms of pure Cidākāśa (pure spiritual space). In the words of the Yoga-vāsiṣṭha:

> "I eulogize that Cidātman who is in that intermediate state when Prāṇa and Apāna are absorbed in one another. I ceaselessly meditate on that Cidātman who is in the Ākāśa directly in front of the root of my nose, when Prāṇa and Apāna become extinct. Thus I attained the Supreme State, worshipped by Devas, through my faultless vision."[22]

Such apotheosis of Bliss and Illumination reaches 'downwards'. Then, there comes neither disease, nor old age, nor death. The 'body' becomes radiant (Deva-like) unto life everlasting. "For God created man to be immortal, and made him to be an image of His own eternity."[23]

The Mudrās, when understood aright, are revealed as a mighty symbol of cosmic proportions. The very symbol of Yoga. Paradoxically, the Mudrās may bring Liberation to the wise but bondage to the fool. For Yoga is the most amazing garden of paradoxes. Without the key to its proper understanding, it is bound to become not a garden, but a veritably impassable jungle to the impure seeker after truth.

Basic Correspondences

Cakra	*Plexus*	*Endocrine Gland*	*Bīja*	*Tattva*	*Conscious level attained, when fully developed*
SAHASRĀRA	OUTER CEREBRAL CORTEX	PINEAL	NĀDA	BUDDHI	SELF-REALIZATION
ĀJÑĀ	CAROTID or CAVERNOUS	PITUITARY	OM	MANAS	WILL CONSCIOUSNESS
VIŚUDDHA	LARYNGEAL	THYROID and PARATHYROIDS	HAṂ	ĀKĀŚA (Ether)	CREATIVE ACTIVITY
ANĀHATA	CARDIAC	THYMUS	YAṂ	VĀYU (Air)	INFINITE COMPASSION
MAṆIPŪRA	SOLAR	SUPRARENALS and PANCREAS	RAṂ	TEJAS (Fire)	SPIRITUAL ASPIRATION
SVĀDHIṢṬHĀNA	SACRAL	OVARIES, TESTES	VAṂ	AP (Water)	TRANSMUTATION/REGENERATION
MŪLĀDHĀRA	COCCYGEAL	COCCYX	LAṂ	PṚTHIVĪ (Earth)	SPIRITUAL AWARENESS

TABLE 1. These Cakras are 'threaded' in the Suṣumnā (core of the Central Nervous System) and form an integral part of a complex threefold-Cakra-System (Etheric, Astral, Mental). For diagrams on the Cakras and other interesting relevant information see 'THE CHAKRAS' and 'MAN VISIBLE AND INVISIBLE' by C.W. Leadbeater, and 'THE SERPENT POWER', by Arthur Avalon.

**Classification of Principles or
Vehicles of Consciousness**

Tāraka Rāja-Yoga	*Vedānta*	*Theosophy*	*Christianity*
ĀTMAN	ĀTMAN	ĀTMIC	SPIRIT
KĀRAṆOPĀDHI (Causal)	ĀNANDAMAYAKOŚA	BUDDHIC VEHICLE	
SŪKṢMOPĀDHI (Subtle)	VIJNĀNAMAYAKOŚA	CAUSAL BODY (Manas)	SOUL
	MANOMAYAKOŚA	MENTAL BODY	
		ASTRAL BODY	
STHŪLOPĀDHI (Gross)	PRĀṆAMAYAKOŚA	ETHERIC	BODY
	ANNAMAYAKOŚA	PHYSICAL	

TABLE 2. Man's subtle anatomy.

The Fourth Lesson

"On account of union with the five sheaths, the pure Ātman appears to be like them, as is the case with a crystal, which appears to be endowed with such colours as blue or red when in contact with a blue or red cloth."

(Ātmabodha, verse 14, by Śri-śaṅkarācārya)

"By complete control over the power of perception it is possible to make outward-turned consciousness inward-turned and become centred in the Ātman, the individualized centre of Reality."

(Śiva-sūtra, III, 12)

PRATYĀHĀRA

(Emotional and Mental Control)

Gheraṇḍa said:

1. Now I shall tell you about the great Pratyāhāra. By such knowledge will all passions like lust, etc. be destroyed.
2. Whenever the Citta (thinking principle) wanders away, attracted by the various objects of sight, bring it back under the control of the Self.
3. When faced with praise or censure, good speech or bad speech, withdraw your mind from all of these and place it under the control of the Self.
4. From sweet smells or bad smells or from whatever odour, withdraw your mind and place it under the control of the Self.
5. From honey-sweet or sour tastes, from bitter or any other by which the mind may be attracted, withdraw it and place it under control of the Self.

This is the shortest lesson in this Yoga treatise, and yet, perhaps it is the one that takes longer to learn: the mastery of the senses or sense-organs, sometimes referred to as the withdrawal of the mind from the objects of sense. Controlling the mind is not something that can be done in one day. It takes enormous patience and skilful know-how. It comes, after perhaps many years of steady practice and wise detachment.

It is noticeable that the writer mentions only four senses: sight, hearing, smell and taste. Obviously, the sense of touch is relatively under our control already, at least in this sense: we may choose to touch something, or to allow ourselves to be touched very much at will. It is true that the rain, for example, may fall upon us and we will most surely feel its impact, but the impacts coming in through the other senses are much more 'volatile', much more subtle, and the psychological reactions they often evoke in us are not so easily warded off. It requires Pratyāhāra. The mind may decide to wander 'out' through the portal of the senses, uncontrolled; or the world may force itself in through those same gateways. In either case one loses Self-control. "The Self is not to be sought through the senses, for these were made facing outwards; therefore, one sees outward and not within oneself. The wise man, seeking life eternal, sees with his eyes turned inwards."[24] Pratyāhāra is the ability of the Yogin to fully detach the mind from the organs of sense and all the psychological conditioning which such sense-dependence implies. Like a tortoise withdrawing its head into its carapace. Such withdrawal is a very subtle, a very skilful thing. It will not help if we simply shut our eyes and ears and block our mouth and nostrils, for in that case, although the world is kept out, the mind remains attached to the inner organs of sense. True Pratyāhāra does not deny, therefore, the senses its free run. What it denies them is the subtle energy of the mind. In that denial there is liberation; in such denial, there is control!

Specific instruction on the performance of Pratyāhāra is, among Yoga treatises, conspicuous by its absence. The Patañjali-yoga-sūtra, in its usually cryptic manner, throws some light in the matter: "Pratyāhāra or abstraction is, as it were, the imitation by the senses of the mind by withdrawing themselves from their objects. Then follows the greatest mastery over the senses."[25] For as long as the mind remains 'connected', attached to even one sense, however lightly, that mind is in worldly bondage and the senses will have full sway, however absorbed that mind may appear to be. It is when the mind is absorbed in itself—reabsorbed—that Pratyāhāra or perfect withdrawal is attained; that point of reabsorption becomes a point without boundaries, a point of perfect control. Pratyāhāra holds the middle ground of Yoga, a point of balance, poised between the outer and the inner. "The absorption of the mind in the Supreme Consciousness by realizing Ātman in all objects is known as Pratyāhāra (withdrawal of the mind) which should be practised by the seekers after liberation."[26] Pratyāhāra does not so much deny the world, as it allows the Yogin to discover its real meaning.

According to a certain tradition, Pratyāhāra can be related to the length of time Prāṇa is fully concentrated in one same place. In higher Yoga, it is claimed that when "the Prāṇa stays in the Brahmarandhra for about 25 Palas (six breaths are called a Pala) that is Pratyāhāra."[27]

The connection between Prāṇa and Mind, and the mastery of

both, is fully discussed in the lessons that follow. In order to approach the gates of liberation, all the other gates must be closed. Hence Pratyāhāra. As the Gītā puts it: "All the gates (sense-organs) closed, the mind confined in the heart, the life-breath (Prāṇa) fixed in his own head, concentrated by Yoga, reciting the one-syllabled Eternal Om meditating upon ME, he who goeth forth, abandoning the body, goeth on the highest path."[28]

Having dealt with Pratyāhāra, the wise Gheraṇḍa next deals with Prāṇāyāma.

The Fifth Lesson

"As the dross of metals is burnt away by the bellows working on the fire, even so all the impurities of the body are consumed and all defects rectified by the controlling and regulating of the breath in the proper ways. To cure physical defects and diseases by breathing exercises; mental diseases and excitements by exercises in concentration of the mind; vicious attachments and addictions of sense by the practice of mental abstraction, and, finally, to overcome the disturbances created by the guṇas of Prakṛti, and all mean and ignoble qualities, by the practice of meditation. The imperishable AUM is the highest Brahman; breath regulation is the highest tapas, ascetic exercise; nothing is higher than the Sāvitrī (Gāyatrī) mantra; than silence Truth is higher."

(Manu, VI, 71-72; II, 83)

PRĀṆĀYĀMA

Gheraṇḍa said:

1. Now I shall give you the correct Prāṇāyāma technique. By its practice one becomes god-like.

The implication of this opening verse is that there exist incorrect practices of Prāṇāyāma, the subject being as much misunderstood as the Mudrās.

2. These things are required, first of all: A good place, a suitable time, regulated nourishment and, finally, the purification of the nāḍīs (subtle channels of prāṇic energy).

The purpose of Prāṇāyāma is twofold: entire harmony and complete mental control. "It is only to control this fickle mind that intelligent Yogins perform Prāṇāyāma. The wise say that the control of Prāṇa leads to that of the mind and causes equality of vision over all. It generates happiness and deters sensual objects from arising in the mind."[29]

A. PLACE

3. This Yoga practice should not be attempted in a distant country, nor in a forest, nor in a capital city surrounded by crowds of people; if one does so, one fails to achieve success.
4. In a distant country, the beginner loses faith; in a forest, one lacks adequate protection; and in the midst of people one exposes oneself to innumerable distractions. Therefore, one should avoid these three.
5. In a good country, under a just government, where plenty of good nourishment is available, free from adversities and distractions, one should erect a small hut encircled by walls.
6. In the centre of such enclosure, one should dig up a well and a cistern. The hut should be neither too high nor too low; let it be free from insects.
7. It should be thoroughly smeared with cow-dung. In such secluded place you should practise Prāṇāyāma.

The important thing to bear in mind here is that the practice of Prāṇāyāma should be carried out in a private place, in safety, with plentiful supplies of adequate food, water and pure and fresh air, amidst pleasant surroundings and sheltered from curious and importunate eyes. Common sense being the hallmark of every true Sādhaka or Yogi-practitioner.

B. TIME

8. This Yoga practice should not begin in any of the following seasons: Winter, early Spring, Summer, or rainy period. If one begins in any of these, one reaps many diseases.
9. The beginner should commence this Yoga practice in Spring or the Autumn. Only so will the Yogin remain free from diseases and achieve adeptship.
10. The seasons occur in their order in the twelve months beginning with Caitra (March) and ending with Phālguna (February), two months to each season. Each season being experienced for four months, beginning with Māgha (January) and ending with Phālguna (February).
11. Spring consists of March and April; Summer, of May and June; Rainy, of July and August; Autumn, of September and October; Winter, of November and December, and Cold, of January and February.
12. Now I shall tell you about the experiencing of the seasons: From January to April we call Spring.
13. From March to June we call Summer; from June to September, Rainy.
14. From August to November, Autumn; from October to January, Winter, and the four months beginning with November, Cold.
15. This Yoga practice should be commenced either in the Spring or the Autumn, for then success is reached without too much exertion.

It is totally inadvisable to begin Prāṇāyāma during the extreme seasons (Summer/Winter) since some of the exercises will prove prejudicial if initially performed in very cold or very hot temperatures, causing a number of inconvenient ills, and upsetting the circulatory and respiratory systems. The intelligent Sādhaka also takes into account the fact that climatic conditions can differ dramatically from region to region.

C. REGULATED NOURISHMENT

16. He who begins this Yoga practice without a regulated diet, reaps various diseases and falls short of success.

The sensible and intelligent Sādhaka ensures that his nourishment is carefully regulated and pure (sattvic). For, as the Bhagavad-gītā expresses it:

> "Men who are pure like food which is pure, which gives health, mental power, strength and long life, which has taste, is soothing and nourishing and which gladdens the heart of man.
> Men of Rajas like food of Rajas: acid and pungent, salty and dry, bringer of heaviness, sickness and pain.
> Men of Tamas eat food which is stale and tasteless, which is rotten and left overnight, impure, unfit for holy offerings."[30]

17. A Yogin should eat rice, barley or wheaten bread, Mudga beans, broad beans, chick peas, etc. These should be clean and free from chaff.
18. He may eat paṭola (a kind of cucumber), jack-fruit, mānakau (Arum Colocasia), kakkola (a kind of berry), the jujube, the bonduc nut (Bonducella guilandina), cucumber, plantain, fig.
19. The unripe plantain, the small plantain, the plantain stem and roots, brinjal, the roots and fruit of the ṛddhi plant.
20. Green, fresh vegetables, black vegetables, the leaves of paṭola, the Vāstūka (a kind of spinach) and himalocikā; these are the five vegetable leaves praised by the Yogins.
21. Pure, sweet and soft food, tasty and pleasant should be eaten to fill half the stomach—this is known as Mītāhāra or regulated nourishment.
22. Half the stomach should be filled with food, one quarter with water; the remainder should be kept empty to allow for free wind movements.
23. In the beginning of this Yoga practice one should abstain from bitter, acid, sour, salty and roasted things; so also

curd, whey, heavy vegetables, alcohol and over-ripe jack-fruit.

24. So also kulattha and masūra beans, pāṇḍu fruit (Trichosanthes dioeca), pumpkins and vegetable stems, gourds, berries, kapittha (Feronia elephantum), kaṇṭa-bilva and palāśa (Butea frondosa).
25. So also kadamba (Nauclea cadamba), jambīra (citron), bimba (Momordica monadelpha), lakuca (a kind of bread fruit tree), garlic, lotus, kāmaraṅga, piyāla (Buchanania latifolia), hiṅgu (assafoetida), śālmali (Salmalia malabarica) and kemuka (Colocasia antiquorum).
26. The beginner should abstain from much travelling, the company of women and warming himself by the fire. He should also avoid fresh butter, ghee, thickened milk, sugar, sugar-cane juice, etc.
27. So also ripe plantain, cocoa-nut, pomegranate, grapes, lavanī fruit (Anona reticulata) and everything containing acid juices.
28. But cardamon, nutmegs, cloves, rose-apple (Eugenia jambolana), jāmbala (Pandanus odoratissimus?) aphrodisiacs, myrobalan (Terminalia chebula) and palm dates, the Yogin may eat during his practice.
29. Easily digestible, enjoyable, tender foods, appropriate to the nourishment of the body, the Yogin may eat to his heart's content.
30. But the Yogin should abstain from not easily digestible, bad or putrid, very hot or very cold as well as stale food.
31. Likewise he should abstain from early morning baths, fasting, etc., or anything injurious to the body, eating only once a day or not eating at all, or remaining without food for more than three hours.

The question of proper, regulated nourishment is vital to the success in Prāṇāyāma. The diet, technically speaking, ought to be 'sattvic' (sweet, pure, wholesome, nourishing and pleasant), otherwise, harmony and free flow of the prāṇic currents through the nāḍīs does not occur, no matter how hard one practises the various prescribed exercises; and Nāda (the inner sound, bestower of success and happiness) remains forever elusive (see Seventh Lesson, 10-11 on Rasānanda-yoga-samādhi). Food should be taken regularly during one's practice and in sufficient quantities. Concentrated sensitivity on this question of nourishment eventually develops an instinct for the proper food and the Sādhaka knows always exactly what, how much and when to take it.

Among the sattvic foods (friends of Prāṇāyāma) one could mention the following representative sample—the list being by no means exhaustive: apples, artichokes, asparagus, apricots, aubergines, bananas, beans, butter, buttermilk, barley, brown and wheaten bread, cabbages, cakes, chick-peas, cauliflowers, currants, cucumbers, carrots, celery, cherries, chestnuts, coconuts, dates, cheese, corn, figs, grapes, ghee, grapefruits, hazelnuts, honey, limes, lentils, lettuce, lemons, macaroni, milk, mandarins, oranges, oats, olives, parsnips, peas, pears, pineapples, potatoes, raisins, peanuts, pomegranates, rice, rye, spinach, strawberries, tomatoes, walnuts.

The enemies of Prāṇāyāma are two-fold: rajasic and tamasic foods. Among the first, we find: coffee, cocoa, fish, garlic, mustard, onions, ovaltine, pepper, radishes, rhubarb, salt and many other. Tamasic foods are: all meats, fried foods, ham, smoked fish, gravies, oysters, pickles, sausages, vinegar, and beverages such as beer, spirits and wines and tobacco, and anything which has been cooked twice (reheated) and anything unclean.

The Prāṇāyāma practitioner is very much a vegetarian and cannot afford not to be one if he really wishes to avoid illness and reach success.

32. Having regulated your life in this manner, you should practise Prāṇāyāma. At first, before commencing your practice, you should take a little milk and ghee daily, twice a day, in the morning and in the evening.

D. PURIFICATION OF NĀḌĪS

33. You should sit on a seat of antelope skin, or tiger skin, or kuśa grass (Poa cynosuroides) or on the ground facing east or north. Having purified the nāḍīs, you should begin Prāṇāyāma.

Caṇḍakāpāli said:

34. Ocean of Compassion! How are the nāḍis purified, what is the purification of the nāḍīs? Tell me, for I am eager to learn.

Gheraṇḍa said:

35. The Vāyu does not enter the nāḍīs so long as they are full of impurities. How, then, can one attain success in Prāṇāyāma? How can there be knowledge of Truth (Tattva-jñāna)? Therefore, one should purify the nāḍīs first; Prāṇāyāma should then be practised.
36. The purification of nāḍīs is either Samanu (with mantra) or Nirmanu (without mantra). Samanu is practised with the help of Bīja-mantra; Nirmanu is performed by physical cleanings.
37. The physical cleanings (Dhautis) have already been described as the six Sādhanas. Listen now, O Caṇḍa, to the Samanu (with mantra) practice.
38. Adopting the lotus posture, the Yogin should first make obeisance to the Guru, etc., as instructed by his teacher; he should then practise the purification of the nāḍīs which brings success in Prāṇāyāma.

Having purified the 'gross' nāḍīs by means of the Dhautis, the Sādhaka is now ready and eager to embark on the purification of the 'subtle' nāḍīs. This purification requires a certain degree of mind control. That is why Pratyāhāra has been described in the previous lesson.

39. Contemplating on Vāyu-bīja (Yaṃ) of a smoke-colour and full of radiance, let the wise Yogin inspire by the Candra-nāḍī (left nostril) repeating the Bīja sixteen times.
40. Let him restrain the breath for a period of sixty-four repetitions of the Bīja-mantra; then, let him expire by the Sūrya-nāḍī (right nostril) whilst repeating the Bīja-mantra thirty-two times.
41. Then, raising the Fire from the Tejas-tattva at the root of the navel, let him contemplate on the blending of it with the Pṛthivī-tattva whilst inspiring by the Sūrya-nāḍī (right nostril) and repeating the Agni-bīja (Raṃ) sixteen times.
42. The breath should be restrained (Kumbhaka) whilst

repeating the Bīja (Raṃ) sixty-four times and then, it should be expired by the Candra-nāḍī (left nostril) whilst repeating the Bīja thirty-two times.

43. Contemplating the luminous radiance of the Moon on the root of the nose, let him inspire by the left nostril repeating the Bīja (Vaṃ) sixteen times.

44. Let him restrain the breath whilst repeating the Bīja (Vaṃ) sixty-four times. At the same time, let him visualize a river of nectar flowing from the Moon and purifying all the nāḍīs; then, whilst repeating the Bīja (Laṃ) thirty-two times let him expire by the Piṅgalā-nāḍī (right nostril) imagining the purification is complete.

The order of purification of the 'subtle' nāḍīs is from Anāhata (Heart-cakra), 'contemplating on Vāyu-bīja (Yaṃ)...', down to the other three cakras, i.e. Maṇipūra, 'by repeating the Agni-bīja (Raṃ)...', Svādhiṣṭhāna, "...repeating the Bīja (Vaṃ), and, finally, Mūlādhāra, or Root-cakra', ...whilst repeating the Bīja (Laṃ). With the lower nāḍīs completely purified by 'the touch of the heart', the Yogin may now move on safely to perform Prāṇāyāma. There is wisdom in beginning one's purification with the Bīja Yaṃ, for, in the words of the Chāndogya Upaniṣad:

> "Verily, these are the three syllables, Sat, Ti, Yaṃ. The Sat, that is the immortal. The Ti, that is the mortal. The Yaṃ, with it one holds the two together. Because with it one holds the two together, therefore, it is Yaṃ. He who knows this goes day by day into the heavenly worlds."[31]

It is only the true Sādhaka who finally discovers the true meaning of Yaṃ, that which holds 'the two' together, the key to Prāṇāyāma.

45. With nāḍīs purified by such a practice, let him adopt a steady posture and perform Prāṇāyāma.

46. Kumbhaka is eightfold: Sahita, Sūryabheda, Ujjāyī, Śītalī, Bhastrikā, Bhrāmarī, Mūrcchā and Kevalī.

1. SAHITA (With in- and out-breathing)

47. Sahita is two-fold: Sagarbha and Nirgarbha. The first is

accompanied by the repetition of Bīja-mantra; the second is not.

48. First I shall instruct you on Sagarbha-prāṇāyāma. Adopting the Sukhāsana* posture, facing east or north, you should contemplate on Brahmā, full of Rajas, red in colour and in the shape of the letter A.

49. Let the wise one inspire by the Iḍā-nāḍī (left nostril) repeating the Bīja (A) sixteen times. Immediately after the end of inhalation, let him perform Uḍḍīyāna-bandha.

50. Then, contemplating on Hari, of a blue colour, full of Sattva quality, let him restrain the breath whilst repeating the Bīja (U) sixty-four times.

51. Then, contemplating on Śiva of a white colour, full of Tamas, let him expire by the right nostril whilst repeating the Bīja (M) thirty-two times.

52. Then, let him inspire by the Piṅgalā (right nostril), restrain the breath by Kumbhaka, and expire by the Iḍā (left nostril) in the same sequential order.

53. This should be repeatedly practised, alternating the nostrils. During Kumbhaka, both nostrils should be closed, the right one by the thumb (of the right hand) and the left one by the little-finger and the ring-finger; never using the index and middle fingers.

The contemplative order of sequence of this delicate and subtle process is from Anāhata-cakra, indicated by the words, 'Brahmā, full of Rajas, red in colour and in the shape of the letter A', to Viśuddha-cakra, 'of a blue colour, full of Sattva quality…', to Ājñā-cakra, the centre of command, the seat of Śiva, where the Bīja 'OM' eternally resides. The emphasis on the positioning of the fingers is to preserve at all times the right 'magnetic' polarity of the extremely subtle energies involved in the process. The reference to 'restraining the breath' ought to be understood in the manner explained at the end of this lesson.

54. The Nirgarbha-(mantraless) prāṇāyāma is practised without repetition of the Bīja. With the palm of the left hand on the left knee, one should control the timing. The period

*'Sukha' means: comfort, pleasure, delight; therefore the text refers to any comfortable posture, preferably cross-legged.

of Pūraka (Inspiration), Kumbhaka (Retention) and Recaka (Expiration) could range from one to a hundred mātrās (seconds).

55. Prāṇāyāma has three levels. The highest (best) is 20; the middle is 16, and the lowest is 12 mātrās.

The ratio of in-breathing, retention and out-breathing is usually given as 1-4-2. Three levels are considered auspicious in the practice of Prāṇāyāma. The author has given us here the middle example, whereby

Inspiration = 16 mātrās
Retention = 64 mātrās
Expiration = 32 mātrās

but, for a proper and correct understanding of the term 'retention", the reader should refer to the end of this lesson, as already indicated.

That this question of Prāṇāyāma is meant to be understood intelligently and not, as it is often the case, too literally, is made absolutely by the following passage attributed to Śrī-saṅkarācārya:

"The negation of the phenomenal world is known as Recaka (expiration), the thought, 'I am verily Brahman', is called Pūraka (inspiration), and the steadiness of that thought thereafter is called Kumbhaka (retention). This is the real course of Prāṇāyāma for the enlightened, whereas the ignorant only torture the nose."[32]

56. The signs of success in the achievement of these three levels of Prāṇāyāma are as follows: by the lowest, the body begins to perspire copiously; practice of the middle causes the body to quiver (especially along the spine); by the highest type, the body leaves the ground (levitation).

57. By Prāṇāyāma one attains Khecarī-siddhi; by Prāṇāyāma all diseases are cured; by Prāṇāyāma, Śakti is awakened; by Prāṇāyāma the mind becomes peaceful and illumined, full of bliss. Blissful is he who practises Prāṇāyāma.

2. SŪRYABHEDA (Pierced by the Sun)

Gheraṇḍa said:

58. I have explained to you the Sahita-kumbhaka; now listen to the Sūryabheda. Inspire vigorously the outer air by the Sūrya-nāḍī (right nostril).

59. Restrain the breath with the utmost care by means of Jālandhara-mudrā and perform the Kumbhaka until the perspiration appears on the tips of the nails and the roots of the hair.

60. Ten are the Vāyus (vital airs), namely: Prāṇa, Apāna, Samāna, Udāna, Vyāna; Nāga, Kūrma, Kṛkara, Devadatta and Dhanañjaya.

61. The Prāṇa moves always in the heart; the Apāna in the anal region; the Samāna in the navel area; the Udāna in the throat and Vyāna throughout the whole body.

62. These are the five principal Vāyus (Prāṇādi); they belong to the interior. The other five begin with Nāga; they belong to the exterior of the body.

63. I now shall tell you the seat of these five outer Vāyus. The Nāga-vāyu causes belching; the Kūrma opens the eye-lids.

64. The Kṛkara causes sneezing; the Devadatta yawning; the Dhanañjaya pervades the whole body and never leaves it, not even after death.

65. The Nāga-vāyu causes (waking) consciousness; the Kūrma gives rise to vision; the Kṛkara, hunger and thirst; the fourth Vāyu (i.e. Devadatta) produces yawning, and by Dhanañjaya sound is produced; this Vāyu does not leave the body even for a second.

66. Draw up all these Vāyus from the root of the navel by the Sūryanāḍī, then, expire by the Iḍā-nāḍī, in a continuous, uninterrupted flow.

67. Once again, inspiring by the right nostril, restrain the breath as instructed and expire again. This should be repeated again and again.

68. The Sūryabheda-kumbhaka conquers old age and death, awakens the Kuṇḍalinī-śakti and fans the gastric fire. O Caṇḍa! Thus have I instructed you on the Sūryabheda-kumbhaka.

3. UJJĀYĪ (Subdued)

69. Inspire the outer air by both nostrils and hold it in the mouth. Draw up the air from the lungs and throat and retain it in the mouth.

70. With mouth so washed and closed, perform Jālandhara-bandha. Kumbhaka should be practised with all one's might without discomfort.

71. All things may be accomplished by Ujjāyī-kumbhaka. One will never be afflicted by phlegm or nerve diseases.

72. Neither dysentery, nor indigestion, nor consumption, nor cough, nor fever, nor enlarged spleen. Practise Ujjāyī-kumbhaka if you desire to conquer old age and death.

4. ŚĪTALĪ (Cooling)

73. Draw in the air through the tongue and fill the stomach (!) slowly. Perform Kumbhaka for a while and expire by both nostrils.

74. A Yogin should constantly practise this Śītalī-kumbhaka; by so doing, he will remain free from indigestion, phlegm and bile disorders.

By 'stomach' is here meant the lower lungs or abdominal region; the air is not to be swallowed but inspired into the lungs, through the rolled tongue.

5. BHASTRIKĀ (Bellows-like)

75. As the bellows of the blacksmith constantly move (expand and contract), so should the Yogin breathe, in and out, by both nostrils.

76. Having thus inspired and expired twenty times, he should perform Kumbhaka. Then, let him expire by the previous method.

77. Let the wise one practise this Bhastrikā-kumbhaka thrice (in succession). He will ever be healthy, free from pain and diseases.

Sūryabheda, Ujjāyī, Śītalī and Bhastrikā are all very powerful and subtle purificatory practices. There is little doubt that, properly carried out, they are of immense physiological and psychological value, and their therapeutic virtues are not to be easily underestimated. They constitute excellent preparation for true Prāṇāyāma.

6. BHRĀMARĪ (Bee-like)

78. After midnight, in a place free from the noise of any creatures, the Yogin should practise Pūraka and Kumbhaka, closing the ears by the hands.
79. He will hear various inner sounds in his right ear. First the sounds will be like that of crickets; then, that of a flute.
80. Then, that of thunder; then, that of a drum; then, that of a beetle; then, that of bells; then, those of gongs, trumpets, trombones, mṛdaṅga, kettle-drums and dundubhi.
81. By steady practice, these various sounds lead finally to the Anāhata sound (Nāda) rising from the heart; of this sound there is a resonance.
82. In that resonance there is a light. In that light the mind should be absorbed. This is the highest seat of Viṣṇu (parama-pada). Success in this Bhrāmarī-kumbhaka leads to success in Samādhi.

The expression 'right ear' ought not to be understood literally; it refers to the 'ear' of the heart. With the progressive purification of the nāḍīs and the steady and increasing mastery of concentration, the Yogin finds it almost natural to achieve progressive levels of Kumbhaka, as a result of which a number of subtle sounds arise out of the body, until, finally, the soundless sound (Anāhata-śabda) or unstruck sound, arises in the heart. As the Voice of the Silence, that priceless gift to theosophical literature, describes it: "He who would hear the voice of Nāda, the soundless sound, and comprehend it, he has to learn the nature of Dhāraṇā."[33] These sounds, although practically innumerable,* form a kind of mystic ladder which is given by that treatise as sevenfold:

> "The first is like the nightingale's sweet voice chanting a song of parting to its mate. The second comes as the sound

*According to Haṃsa Upaniṣad, for example, ten sorts of such sounds are experienced by the yogin.

of a silver cymbal of the Dhyanis, awakening the twinkling stars. The next is as the plaint melodious of the ocean-sprite imprisoned in its shell. And this is followed by the chant of Vīṇā. The fifth like sound of bamboo-flute shrills in thy ear. It changes next into a trumpet blast. The last vibrates like the dull rumbling of a thunder cloud. The seventh swallows all the other sounds. They die, and then are heard no more."[34]

These blissful sounds arise from the void (Śūnya) in the heart (Anāhata) and, following the upward and secret path, uninterrupted, like a fine and steady flow of oil, the peal of a continuous sound, the Prāṇa enters the middle void (Atiśūnya) and, later, the great void (Mahāśūnya), the sphere of Ājñā-cakra, which is the seat of all perfection. In that space, full of resonance, there is a light, the light of the Self. In that light, the mind finds peace and liberation.

Needless to say, the above description refers to success not merely in Prāṇāyāma but in Yoga, and it represents a very advanced stage in the Sādhaka's practice.

7. MŪRCCHĀ (Fainting)

83. Having performed Kumbhaka with comfort, let him withdraw the mind from all sense objects and fix it in the space between the eye-brows. This causes fainting of the mind and bestows happiness. By the union of Manas with the Ātman, spiritual Bliss is certainly attained.

This Mūrcchā is an elaborate form of Śāmbhavī-mudrā whereby the important role played by Prāṇāyāma is indicated. In the advanced stages of Yoga practice, Kumbhaka occurs naturally, almost spontaneously and without effort. Hence the expression 'with comfort'—as a result of the perfect union of Ha (Śiva) and Ṭha (Śakti) and not by means of Haṭha (forceful) Yoga. In such natural union, there is immense happiness and spiritual Bliss; one no longer breathes: one is Breath. Breath is all there is.

8. KEVALĪ (Whole)

84. With the sound 'Saḥ' the breath goes in; with the sound 'Haṃ' the breath comes out—twenty-one thousand and

six hundred times every 24 hours. Every living being (Jīva) performs this Ajapā Gāyatrī unconsciously and continuously.

85. This Ajapā-japa is performed in three places: in Mūlādhāra, in the heart lotus (Anāhata) and where the nostrils meet (Ājñā).

These three places (knots or granthis, as they are often referred to) are the intersecting points of Iḍā (Saḥ = Śakti = Moon) and Piṅgalā (Haṃ = Śiva - Sun). The word 'Soham' (He am I) is pronounced by a deep inspiration followed by expiration carried on by the nostrils. This Ajapā Gāyatrī, normally offered unconsciously, is what the Yogin learns to offer consciously. The proper technique consists in making such offering by 'pronouncing' the mantra in 'reverse', offering the out-breathing in the in-breathing, and vice-versa.

86. The body is on average 96 digits (six feet) long. The ordinary (natural) length of the expired current (of air) is 12 digits (9 inches).

87. In singing, its length is 16 digits (one foot); in eating it is 20 digits (15 inches); in walking, it is 24 digits (18 inches); in sleep, it is 30 digits (22½ inches); in copulation, it is 36 digits (27 inches) and in taking physical exercise, even more than that.

88. By decreasing the ordinary (natural) length of the expired current from 12 digits to less, there comes increase of life; by increasing the current, there is decrease of life.

A forcible expiration is always considered a sign of loss, dissolution, perhaps even death. The text refers to the disadvantages (decrease of life) incurred by the lengthening of the expired air current. What of the opposite? What, then, can one say about shortening (decreasing) the length of the expired air current? It is the view of certain Yoga tradition that when it is reduced to 6 inches, one acquires the power of foretelling the future; reduction to 4½ inches enables one to travel through space; a further reduction allows the Yogin to embrace the whole wide world in the twinkling of an eye, etc. It is written, in the Yoga-vāsiṣṭha that,

"If the motion of Prāṇa and therefore the mind be arrested both internally and externally, then death and dotage fly to a great distance."[35]

Like everything else one finds in most—if not all—Yoga treatises, one will be well advised not to take things too literally. It is true that the process of Prāṇāyāma is a vital one, fundamentally important to Yoga, and that it has even been claimed that the various stages of Yoga are simply stages of Prāṇāyāma, but the question remains, what is Prāṇāyāma? and, what is Kevalī?

Our final commentary will attempt to answer both these questions.

89. For as long as breath abides in the body, there is no death. When the full length of the breath is confined within the body, this is Kevala-kumbhaka.
90. All living beings are constantly and unconsciously repeating this Ajapā-mantra for a fixed number of times daily.
91. But the Yogin should perform this Ajapā-japa consciously. By doubling the number of Ajapā (i.e. by 30 respirations per minute instead of 15) the mind becomes peaceful and illumined (Manonmanī).

Here the text, at last, spells out the technique of Kevala-kumbhaka. Needless to say, the mere doubling of the respirations per minute in order to attain success in Prāṇāyāma is far too simple a technique and it is not to be understood literally, as it is often the case. It would be extremely naive to do so. The meaning of this verse will be made clear with our final commentary.

92. Having inspired the air by both nostrils, let him perform Kevala-kumbhaka. On the first day, the breath should be retained from one to sixty-four times.
93. Perform this Kevalī once every Yāma (three hours) or five times a day, as I shall tell you.
94. In the early morning, at noon, in the evening, at midnight and then, in the fourth quarter of the night. Or, thrice a day: in the morning, noon and evening.
95. The length of Ajapā-japa should be increased everyday, from one to five times, until success (siddhi) is achieved.

96. For him who knows Yoga, Prāṇāyāma is Kevalī. What can he not accomplish on this earth who has achieved mastery in Kevala-kumbhaka?

We have come now to the end of the Fifth Lesson on Prāṇāyāma. For 'him who knows Yoga', Prāṇāyāma is Kevalī, and vice-versa. What is Prāṇāyāma?

Very often, the term is found translated as meaning control of the breath (Prāṇa-yama) which has the sense of effort and restrain; whereas a better and more accurate translation would be to consider the word as the result of two other words, Prāṇa and āyāma, where the second term means to extend, to expand, to lengthen—both in time and space. What is it, then, that should be expanded, lengthen? The interval, the gap between in-breathing out-breathing. It is because of this, that the Bhagavadgītā, in referring to the various types of sacrifice offered by Yogins, states:

> "...Yet others pour as sacrifice the outgoing breath in the incoming, and the incoming in the outgoing, restraining the flow of the outgoing and incoming breaths, solely absorbed in the control of breathing."[36]

Thus revealing, in part, the true nature of Prāṇāyāma. It isn't always easy to understand the exact meaning of such words because the process involves a subtle extension into a different kind of space; a very gradual transit from a gross activity to a subtle one. It implies a going beyond the boundaries of in- and out-breathing, increasing one's awareness of the interval and very gradually lengthening and refining the in-breathing and the out-breathing until they both 'meet each other', in the most subtle of embraces, so that one can hardly tell which one is going out and which one is coming in, in perfect union (Ha-ṭha). And to dissolve later in a point of infinitesimal Bliss. In the words of G.S. Arundale:

> "Within what may be called limitless contraction there is infinitude no less than within the limitless expansion with which we are much more accustomed to associate the idea of infinitude. In that Ceaseless Breath of God, ... we conceive of an infinitude of out-breathing and equally, of an infinitude of in-breathing..."[37]

He who has mastered Kevalī, has mastered the Rhythm of infinitude. He has come to Yoga.

Patañjali, in a few masterly aphorisms, helps us to elucidate the subject even further:

> "Āsana having been perfected, Prāṇāyāma (cessation of the boundary between inspiration and expiration) follows. It is external, internal or steady; regulated by place, time and number; and is long and subtle.
> The fourth is that which has no bearing on the external and internal positions."[38]

The breath (Prāṇa) having now become so subtle that, although still mysteriously abiding in the body, it really knows no abiding place. True Prāṇāyāma enables the Yogin to attain supreme harmony and perfect equilibrium of the Prāṇic system, so that he may, at last, be able to control his 'fickle mind', as the Yoga-vāsiṣṭha says. This complex Prāṇic system operates in terms of a threefold polarity:

Iḍā (left, Moon)	and Piṅgalā (right, Sun)
Up (Prāṇa)	and Down (Apāna)
In (Saḥ)	and Out (Haṃ)

The meeting point of all these, when perfectly harmonized, is Kevala-kumbhaka, the crown of Prāṇāyāma. It is a point where movement and rest co-exist in perfect equilibrium. In the words of a modern Yogin:

> "... For us the Rhythm or Law of the Ceaseless Breath is surely not only one of the ultimates, but perchance even the Ultimate. I shall not hesitate to say that it is the Rhythm both of movement and movementlessness. It is the substance of THAT. Where Rhythm is stilled to its uttermost, is at its slowest, there remains Ceaseless Breath, even though the vacuum seems almost complete. Where Rhythm is infinitely vibrant, there is the Ceaseless Breath."[39]

Now, from the more intuitional to the more practical. It is common knowledge that, at times, one nostril seems to be freer than the other; later, the somewhat 'stuffed' nostril suddenly becomes freer, and it is the other nostril which in turn becomes partially blocked. This process alternates with regularity (approximately every two hours). Nature follows a certain inner rhythm, in terms of 'right' and 'left'. Then, sometimes, our in-breathing takes longer than our out-breathing, or vice-versa. Sometimes we breathe noisily; at times, we breathe so gently that even we hardly notice we are breathing; sometimes, quite suddenly, we realize that, for a moment, we have stopped breathing altogether and avidly gasp for breath.

The purpose of Prāṇāyāma is to introduce harmony and rhythm into such irregular performance, so that one may attain to a greater harmony. If the breath wanders irregularly, how can anyone ever hope to acquire a steady mind? That is why the breath must be balanced. First, 'right' and 'left' must be purified, equilibrated (Sahita, Sūryabheda). Then, proficiency in Kumbhaka and concentration, pursued with effortless diligence, ensures the balance of 'up' and 'down', and 'in' and 'out'. Effort should play no part in Prāṇāyāma, for this is the gentlest of all arts: the supreme art of Life; and the intense, clear, deepening awareness of life is found in the 'pause' between in-breathing and out-breathing, the mysterious interval of Ha-ṭha Yoga. In the experience of that pause, there is peace; the mind then becomes very silent, and out of that deep silence, "...the mysterious event will occur which will prove that the way has been found."[40] As Patañjali puts it, "Thence is destroyed the covering of the light, and the mind becomes fit for contemplation."[41] It is this 'fitness' of the mind that the intelligent practitioner aspires to. Prāṇāyāma, when properly understood, gradually leads to Rāja-yoga and Liberation.

The Yogavāsiṣṭha provides a few more helpful directions towards the correct understanding of this difficult subject:

> "In the cool lotus of the heart within this visible tenement of flesh composed of the five elements, there are two Vāyus, Prāṇa and Apāna, mingled in it...These Vāyus go up and down to higher and lower states. They have the same nature in the waking, dreaming and dreamless sleeping states, and permeate all. Divide a filament of the lotus stalk a thousand times and you will find these Vāyus more subtle than that...Of these, Prāṇa ceaselessly vibrates in this body with an upward motion, both externally and

internally, while Apāna, having the same fluctuating tendency, vibrates both external and internal to the body, having a downward motion. It is beneficial if the Prāṇa exhaled (to the extent of sixteen digits) is inhaled to the same extent. Those who have brought to experience this (i.e. equalization of Prāṇa in exhalation and inhalation) will enjoy infinite bliss."[42]

The importance of Prāṇāyāma is due to the fact that Prāṇa and Mind are closely related to each other. The correspondences between Prāṇa and Mind, from the point of view of Yoga practice, are as follows:

i. The rhythmically balanced breath normally accompanies the stage of Pratyāhāra. It is sometimes referred to as the pendular breath (Tāla-yukta).
ii. When the breath becomes 'uninterrupted', fully extended, lengthened, continuous (the out-breathing in the in-breathing and vice-versa); this is a sign of a deeply concentrated mind (Dhāraṇā). The breath is fully expanded-confined 'within the body'. This is the initial stage of Kevala-kumbhaka.
iii. A further stage of Kevala-kumbhaka is reached when the breath becomes gradually shorter and subtler; the in-breathing and the out-breathing getting 'closer to each other'; earlier, they had merged, now they fuse together in 'passionate embrace'. This stage accompanies the various stages of Meditation (Dhyāna) and is the real meaning behind the expression found in verse 91, where the Yogin is expected to, consciously, 'double the number of Ajapā, i.e. from 15 to 30 per minute!'
iv. The total and perfect union (Laya) of in-breathing and out-breathing (Apāna-Prāṇa/Saḥ-Haṃ) finally indicates (not, produces) the presence of the stage of Samādhi, when the knower, the knowledge and the known are experienced as one.

One could be tempted to say that the stages of Pratyāhāra, Dhāraṇā, Dhyāna and Samādhi, are simply stages of Prāṇāyāma, gradually increasing in subtleness. Such conclusion would be too simplistic and would indicate a complete misunderstanding of the true nature of Yoga. It was, no doubt, the closeness of such relationship between Prāṇa and Mind that led Śri-śaṅkarācārya to claim that "the restraint of all modifications of the mind by regarding all mental states like the Citta as Brahman alone, is called Prāṇāyāma."[43]

The Sixth Lesson

"All the gates (sense organs) closed, the mind confined in the heart, the life-breath (Prāṇa) fixed in his own head, concentrated by Yoga, reciting the one-syllabled Eternal Om meditating upon ME, he who goeth forth, abandoning the body, goeth on the highest path."

(Bhagavadgītā, VIII, 12-13)

DHYĀNA-YOGA

Gheraṇḍa said:

1. There are three kinds of Dhyāna (Meditation): gross, luminous and subtle. The first is directed to physical figures or shapes (Sthūla); the second has light (Jyotis) for support; the third is fixed on Brahman as Bindu (Sūkṣma) and the Goddess Kuṇḍalinī.

In the same way as one may talk about man as consisting of Body, Soul and Spirit, one can approach the question of Meditation in the manner chosen by Gheraṇḍa: a threefold treatment in which Sthūla=Body, Jyotis=Soul, and Bindu=Spirit; or gross, luminous and subtle. Using the Lotus symbol, one could compare these three levels to 'roots, stem and petals'. For an understanding of various possible methods of classification, the reader will find it interesting to study Tables 1 and 2. Gheraṇḍa's approach, allowing for slight differences in terminology, corresponds very closely to the Tāraka Rāja-yoga system.

1. STHŪLA DHYĀNA

2. Let him picture a large ocean of nectar in the region of the heart and in the midst of that ocean an island of precious stones, the sand itself being of finest gems.
3. On the four sides of it, kadamba trees, in full bloom, and next to those trees, like a rampart, a row of flowering trees.
4. Mālati, mallikā, jāti, kesara, campaka, pārijāta and padma, spreading beautiful fragrance in all directions.
5. In the middle of this garden, let the Yogin imagine a beautiful kalpa tree, having four branches, symbolizing the four Vedas, full of flowers and fruits.
6. The bees are humming and the cuckoos are calling there. Beneath that tree, let him imagine a rich platform of rubies and other precious gems.
7. Let the Yogin imagine, on this rich platform, a sumptuous

throne inlaid with jewels, and that on that throne sits his Iṣṭa-devatā (chosen Deity), as taught to him by his Guru.

8. Let him meditate on the form of this Deity (symbolic ornaments and vehicle). The steady meditation on such a form, is Sthūla Dhyāna.

Having found the way to the Heart (with Heart purified) with the help of Prāṇāyāma, the Yogin, now swimming in the ocean of nectar, is enabled to reach the promised land (island), the dwelling of the beloved (Iṣṭa-devatā). The purpose in providing such a colourful and detailed symbol for meditation, is to lessen the initial difficulty of the mind to remain confined within a limited 'mental' area for a long period of time; the mind, normally, tends to wander with extreme rapidity, almost unnoticed, from one thing to another; in the words of the Gītā, "...the mind is hard to curb and restless; but it may be curbed by constant practice and dispassion (non-attachment)."[44] So difficult is it to control, in fact, that a text like the Kūrma Purāṇa maintains that should the mind remain fully concentrated for only 12 seconds the stage of Dhāraṇā is reached; twelve times that period produces Dhyāna, and, in turn, twelve times that, Samādhi. The idea of this meditation is to allow the mind enough free movement to search for the beloved within the suggested limited mental area, so that it does not wander away altogether. The 'technique' is perfectly scientific, and more than one scientist or investigator approach their research—if they are really serious—with very much the same attitude or frame of mind, and perhaps equal devotion.

In seeking union, the Yogin may choose to search for the beloved 'in the Heart', or 'in the Head'; these being the Self's two favourite residing places. That this is so, the method that follows makes absolutely clear.

1a. ANOTHER METHOD

9. You should imagine that in the pericarp of the great thousand-petalled Lotus (Sahasrāra-padma), there is a smaller lotus having twelve petals.

10. Its colour is white, radiant with light, and having twelve

Bīja letters, as follows: ha, sa, kṣa, ma, la, va, ra, yuṃ, ha, sa, kha, phreṃ.

11. In the centre of the pericarp of this smaller lotus there are three lines forming a triangle A-Ka-Tha with angles Ha-La-Kṣa. In the centre of this triangle abides the Praṇava 'OM'.
12. Then let him picture in its centre a beautiful seat having Nāda and Bindu, and on it, a pair of wooden sandals and two swans.
13. There let him meditate on Gurudeva, having two arms and three eyes, dressed in pure white, and anointed with white sandal-paste.
14. Wearing garlands of white flowers, with Śakti of blood-red colour beside him. By thus meditating on the Guru, Sthūla Dhyāna is attained.

The symbology of this meditation points in the direction of the complex system formed by the Medulla Oblongata and the Pituitary and Pineal glands, the mystic triangle (▽). The Praṇava 'OM' being the Bīja mantra of Ājñā-cakra, as indicated earlier (V, 51). It is here that the 'unstruck sound', Nāda, reigns supreme. "O, the process of incessantly hearing Nāda! I bow down to you. I consider you as the worthiest of all the means for the absorption of the mind. For, through your grace, my mind along with the vital breath gets absorbed in Viṣṇu-pada, i.e. the 'sky' which is that absolute Supreme of the nature of Saccidānanda."[45] So wrote Śrīśaṅkarācārya near the end of his days.

That the Medulla Oblongata is involved would seem reasonable to assume, since it contains the controlling centres for the heartbeat and respiration But on no account should the Sādhaka ever attempt to influence the Medulla directly, for the most disastrous effects would surely follow, without a doubt. In true meditation, the breath remains controlled always from 'above', so to speak.

2. JYOTIR-DHYĀNA

Gheraṇḍa said:

15. I have explained to you the Sthūla Dhyāna; hear now

about the meditation on the Light, by which the Yogin attains to Siddhi and knowledge of the Self.

16. In the Mūlādhāra is Kuṇḍalinī of the form of a snake. The Jīvātman is there like the point of a flame. Meditate on this flame as the luminous Brahman. This is the even greater Light-meditation.

2a. ANOTHER METHOD

17. In the middle of the eye-brows, above the Manas, there is the light of 'OM'. Meditate on this Light as if surrounded by flames. This is another form of contemplation of the Light.

Success in Sthūla Dhyāna, leads to luminous meditation, meditation on the light of the Self. Every object has a distinct counterpart of light. By deepening one's meditation, one learns to commune with the soul (light) of the object meditated upon; in this particular case, the light of 'OM'. The symbology of this meditation is much more austere than the previous one; there is nothing sophisticated here to entrance, to hold the mind, but a pure, naked flame, the object of one's search. "As a lamp in a windless place flickereth not, to such is likened the Yogin of subdued thought, absorbed in the Yoga of the Self."[46] At last, the light is seen, and one comes to knowledge of the Self. This stage is accompanied by the advanced stage of Kevalī, whereby, as Patañjali says, "is destroyed the covering of the light."[47]

By meditation on the light, the Yogin attains to Siddhi. "Knowledge of the small, the hidden or the distant, by directing the light of superphysical faculty."[48] This Light-meditation, if carried out successfully, augurs well for the activation of the Suṣumnā mechanism and the awakening of Kuṇḍalinī-śakti, and, therefore, the Sādhaka also experiences a blissful heat arising from the Mūlādhāra region, where the Golden Kuṇḍalinī, guardian of the Flame, resides; and without whose help no real ascent in Yoga is ever possible. To quote from the Christian Gospels:

> "And no man hath ascended up to heaven, but he that came down from heaven, even the Son of man which is in heaven.

And as Moses lifted up the serpent in the wilderness, even so must the Son of man be lifted up:
That whosoever believeth in him should not perish, but have Eternal Life."[49]

Which, esoterically understood simply means that Kuṇḍalinī must be lifted up; the Son of man (Jīvātman) also must be lifted up. True, pure Yoga consists in fully understanding and experiencing this lifting up.

Of this Suṣumnā mechanism, whereby such awakening is made possible, it has been said that,

> "The Trans-Himālayan School. . .locates Suṣumnā, the chief seat of these three Nāḍīs, in the central tube of the spinal cord; and Iḍā and Piṅgalā on its left and right side. Suṣumnā is the Brahmadaṇḍa. . .Iḍā and Piṅgalā are simply the sharps and flats of that Fa of human nature. . .which, when struck in a proper way, awakens the sentries on either side, the spiritual Manas and the physical Kāma, and subdues the lower through the higher. But this effect has to be produced by the exercise of will-power,* not through the scientific or trained suppression of the breath."[50]

This meditation awakens the will and, as the text claims, is a hundred times superior to the previous one. The meditation which follows, however, is even far superior.

3. SŪKṢMA DHYĀNA

Gheraṇḍa said:

18. O Caṇḍa! You have heard about Light-meditation. Listen now to the Sūkṣma Dhyāna. When by some blissful grace, Kuṇḍalinī awakes.
19. It joins the Ātman and, travelling together, leaves the body through the portals of the eyes, treading the Royal Path. It defies perception, however, because of its evasive and subtle form.

*By 'will-power', the writer refers here to the active Spiritual Will, the sphere of Ājñā-cakra. Iḍā and Piṅgalā corresponding to the autonomic and Suṣumnā to the central nervous system.

20. The Yogin, however, attains to success by means of Śāmbhavī-mudrā. This is the mysteriously subtle meditation (Sūkṣma Dhyāna) difficult of attainment, even by the Devas.

Kuṇḍalinī-śakti (the Golden Serpent, the Fire Vestal), joining the spiritual Self (Ātman) in subtle embrace, sets off on her nuptial journey from Mūlādhāra to Ājñā-cakra Here, 'leaving the body through the portals of the eyes', from Ājñā to Sahasrāra, together, they tread the Royal Path (the path of Rāja-yoga). The process is an extremely subtle one, impossible to put into words and has little, if anything, to do with the physical body; hence the reference to 'it defies perception'. The Yogin requires to give his total attention to this delicate inner experience, hence it is recommended that he practises Śāmbhavī-mudrā. This allows for the blissful vision of the Flame (tongue) being swallowed up, and which, eventually, leads to the union of Ātman with Paramātman, the goal of Samādhi. This meditation gives birth to the 'Third Eye'; the eye that never slumbers or sleeps, faithfully guarding the City of the Seven Gates:

> "And the city had no need of the Sun, neither of the Moon, to shine in it: for the Glory of God did lighten it, and the Lamb is the light thereof. And the gates of it shall not be shut at all by day, for there shall be no night there."[51]

This meditation also unveils for us the real meaning of Khecarī-mudrā.

21. The meditation on Light is a hundred times superior to meditation on Form; and a hundred thousand times superior to Tejodhyāna is meditation on the Sūkṣma.
22. O Caṇḍa! Thus have I portrayed for you the extremely arduous path of Meditation (Dhyāna)—a most precious knowledge; for it leads to the direct perception of the Self. Hence its constant praise.

A most vivid psychophysiological illustrative description of these advanced stages in meditation is given in The Secret Doctrine:

"We begin with the mastery of that organ which is situated at the base of the brain, in the pharynx, and called by Western anatomists the Pituitary Body. In the series of objective cranial organs, corresponding to the subjective Tattvic principles, it stands to the Third Eye (Pineal Gland) as Manas stands to Buddhi; the arousing and awakening of the Third Eye must be performed by that vascular organ, that insignificant little body, of which, once again, Physiology knows nothing at all. The one is the energizer of Will, the other that of Clairvoyant Perception...
When a man is in his normal condition, an Adept can see the golden Aura pulsating in both centres, like the pulsation of the heart, which never ceases throughout life. This motion, however, under the abnormal condition of effort to develop clairvoyant faculties, becomes intensified, and the Aura takes on a stronger vibratory or swinging action. The arc of the pulsation of the Pituitary Body mounts upward, more and more, until, just as when the electric current strikes some solid object, the current finally strikes the Pineal Gland, and the dormant organ is awakened and set all glowing with the pure Ākāśic Fire. This is the psychophysiological illustration of two organs on the physical plane, which are, respectively, the concrete symbols of the metaphysical concepts called Manas and Buddhi. The latter, in order to become conscious on this plane, needs the more differentiated fire of Manas; but once the sixth sense has awakened the seventh, the light which radiates from this seventh sense illumines the fields of infinitude. For a brief space of time man becomes omniscient; the Past and the Future, Space and Time, disappear and become to him the Present. If an Adept, he will store the knowledge he thus gains in his physical memory, and nothing, save the crime of indulging in Black Magic, can obliterate the remembrance of it. If only a Chelā, portions alone of the whole truth will impress themselves on his memory, and he will have to repeat the process for years, never allowing one speck of impurity to stain him mentally or physically, before he becomes a fully initiated Adept."[52]

The above description refers to the stages of Rāja-yoga proper, for a fuller elaboration of which one must seek the assistance of a fully enlightened and trustworthy guru; no easy thing to achieve at the best of times. Texts such as the Patañjali-yoga-sūtra will also prove of inestimable value to the sincere and discriminating Sādhaka. In dealing with Meditation, Patañjali has provided us with the general guidelines:

> "Uninterrupted flow (of the mind) towards the object (chosen for meditation) is contemplation.
> The same (contemplation) when there is consciousness only of the object of meditation and not of itself (the mind) is Samādhi."[53]

All success in Yoga depends on this 'uninterrupted flow', this perfect continuity of aspiration, this constantly 'pulsating upward' movement from the unreal to the Real; from darkness to Light; from death to Immortality and Perfect Liberation, the goal of Samādhi.

Some correspondences in the Haṭha/Rāja-Yoga System: MEDITATION

Āsana	*Mudrā*	*Prāṇāyāma*	*Breathing Ratios* (*In* | *Pause* | *Out*)	*Centre*	*Symbol*	*Stage*
VAJRĀSANA	TRĀṬAKA	RHYTHMIC (Pendular)	LONG—SHORT—LONG	OBJECT	LIGHT	PRATYĀHĀRA
SIDDHĀSANA	ŚĀMBHAVĪ	KEVALĪ I	LONG—LONG—LONG (Uninterrupted-Expanded: "Inbreating in Outbreathing."	EYE-BROWS	SUN-DISC (ANĀHATA-ŚABDA)	DHĀRAṆĀ
SIDDHĀSANA	KHECARĪ I	KEVALĪ II	SHORT—SHORT—SHORT Imperceptible—"Inpanded")	PITUITARY	FLAME-NĀDA	DHYĀNA
PADMĀSANA	KHECARĪ II	LAYA	SUBTLE (LATENT) Breathing through "a point" (Bindu)	PINEAL	SELF IN THE FLAME (SOUND)	SAMĀDHI

TABLE 3. The āsanas given here are only indicative and represent the author's own personal choice.

The Seventh Lesson

"Lord! whose Real nature is expressed in the manifested universe as Divine Consciousness and Power, be pleased to remove this outer veil so that my constant remembrance and devotion towards Thee may find consummation in my direct perception of Thy Real Nature within my heart."

(Īśāvāsya Upaniṣad, mantra 15)

SAMĀDHI-YOGA

Gheraṇḍa said:

1. Finally, Samādhi is a greater Yoga; it is the result of good fortune (Karma). It is obtained by the kindness and grace of the Guru, and by intense devotion to Him.
2. This splendid practice of Samādhi is quickly attained by the Yogin who has trust in the teaching and faith in the Guru and his own Self, and whose mind awakens from day-to-day.
3. Separate the thinking principle (Manas) from the body, and unite it with Paramātman. This is known as Ecstasy (Samādhi) or Mukti, liberation from all states of consciousness.
4. I am Brahman (the Absolute) and nothing else; verily am I Brahman and sorrow is not my lot. My nature is Pure Existence, Consciousness and Bliss (Saccidānanda), eternally free, the only true Self.

The expression, 'by the kindness and grace of the Guru', refers to the mysteries of Initiation and the arousal of Kuṇḍalinī, and it is often 'exoterically' interpreted as meaning the act of intercession by one's master by means of his hand-touch, the use of certain prescribed mantras appropriate to the particular occasion, a glance, or even his mere wish. As it is written in the Śiva-sūtra:

> "The Spiritual Teacher who initiates the disciple does this by uniting the consciousness of the disciple with his own and giving him direct knowledge of Mātṛkā-cakra, through which the power of 'sound' descends into manifestation."[54]

Needless to say, the real Guru is also one's Higher Self, the Ātman, or 'the Puruṣa of the size of a thumb', as the Upaniṣads often described Him, forever dwelling in the 'cave of the Heart'. For, as the Voice of the Silence so aptly and poetically puts it:

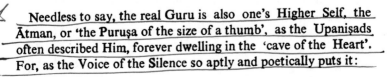

> "The light from the One Master, the one unfading golden light of Spirit, shoots its effulgent beams on the disciple from the very first. Its rays thread through the thick dark clouds of matter. Now here, now there, these rays illumine it, like sun-sparks light the earth through the thick foliage of the jungle growth. But, O Disciple, unless the flesh is passive, head cool, the soul as firm and pure as flaming diamond, the radiance will not reach the chamber, its sunlight will not warm the heart, nor will the mystic sounds of the Ākāśic heights reach the ear, however eager at the initial stage."[55]

The state of Samādhi transcends the three other states of consciousness, traditionally known as Jāgrat (waking), Svapna (dreaming) and Suṣupti (dreamless sleep). Thus it is referred to as Turīya (the fourth). These three states correspond in a mysterious way to the three kinds of Dhyāna examined earlier, Sthūla, Jyotis and Sūkṣma, which refer to awareness of inner processes and the inner planes of vibration or manifestation, i.e. etheric, astral, mental. In Samādhi, however, the Yogin transcends the mental plane altogether, 'the thinking principle (Manas) separated from the body and firmly united with Paramātman', as the text puts it. Success in Sūkṣma-dhyāna confers upon the Yogin a certain degree of union and mastery over the world of manifestation. The next step, Samādhi is intended to bring him to union with Īśvara, the Creator, the Supreme embodiment of Divine Wisdom, Brahman, Saccidānanda, his very true Self; however one chooses to describe it. Little by little, through Purification (Cleansings, Āsanas, Prāṇāyāma), the establishment of harmony by mastering the organs of sense (Pratyāhāra), achievement of perfect harmony within (Kevalī), and constant, uninterrupted, spiritual aspiration (various stages of Dhyāna), plus the graceful intercession of the 'Guru', the Yogin manages to extricate himself from the worlds of illusion (the realms of his infinitely complex 'anatomy'). With consciousness forever reaching upward (inwards), he finally approaches the deepest mystery, the very source of his being, his very true Self.

Two mystic elements guide the Yogin in these final stages: Light and Sound. For,

"Unless thou hearest, thou canst not see.
Unless thou seest, thou canst not hear."[56]

This ascent to the peaks of Samādhi is often accompanied by certain unmistakable signs, the nature of which can even, at times, puzzle the unenlightened Sādhaka. In the words of G.S. Arundale, one experiences,

> "a mystic thunder and lightning wholly comparable to its physical counterpart...And so far as my own experiences attest, there is a certain form of Yoga, some of the higher reaches of which seem to have a setting of semi-cosmic thunder and of lightning, so that the appellation gained by St. John of 'Son of Thunder' is that of all who have attained such regions."[57]

These two elements, Light and Sound, end eventually, in that which is soundless, the highest state of Samādhi. To quote from the Book of Revelation:

> "And when he had opened the seventh seal, there was silence in heaven about the space of half an hour."[58]

In such Silence there is Truth.

5. Samādhi is fourfold: Dhyāna, Nāda, Rasānanda and Laya-siddhi, respectively attained by Śāmbhavī-mudrā, Khecarī-mudrā, Bhrāmarī-kumbhaka and Yoni-mudrā.
6. The Bhakti-yoga-samādhi is fifth, and Rāja-yoga-samādhi, attained through Mano-mūrcchā-kumbhaka, is the sixth.

restraining movement of mind!

1. DHYĀNA-YOGA SAMĀDHI

7. Perform the Śāmbhavī-mudrā and perceive the Ātman. Meditating on Bindu as Brahman, fix the mind on that luminous point.
8. Place the Ātman in Kha (Ether), and Kha in the Ātman. Thus, seeing the Ātman full of Kha, nothing will obstruct him. Perfectly blissful, the Yogin enters Samādhi.

The word Bindu here means solar disc or shining point. Dhyāna-yoga-samādhi has for 'support' the Light element, the

'I' consciousness shining in the midst of the Pituitary/Pineal body complex. Śāmbhavī-mudrā ensures that the awareness is directed as a constant, effortless flow to the right spot, commonly known as the space between the eye-brows, in mystical contemplation of the luminous Ātman. In the words of the Īśa Upaniṣad,

> "The door of the Truth is covered by a golden disc. Open it, O Nourisher! Remove it so that I who have been worshipping the Truth may behold it."[59]

The expression, 'O Nourisher', refers to Kuṇḍalinī-śakti. And, drawing upon the inspirational wisdom of the Gītā,

> "Having external contacts excluded, and with gaze fixed between the eye-brows; having made equal the outgoing and ingoing breaths moving within the nostrils; with senses, Mind and Buddhi ever controlled, solely pursuing liberation, the sage, having forever cast away desires, fear and passion, verily is liberated."[60]

2. NĀDA-YOGA-SAMĀDHI

9. By performing Khecarī-mudrā, with the tongue turned upwards, Samādhi is reached. (Achieving this) all other practices are superfluous.

Nāda-yoga-samādhi also has for 'support' both the Light and Sound elements. As the reader already knows by now, this stage is reached not by swallowing one's tongue till it reaches the spot between the eye-brows, as the word Khecarī is usually interpreted and which is the hallmark of Jaḍa (stone and therefore false) Samādhi; but by the union of the individual Soul (Ha) with Śiva (Ṭha), the Self to the SELF united in flaming embrace; the flaming embrace at Golgotha[61]—the place of the skull—the Christ Centre. It is called Nāda-yoga because it is a roaring embrace, full of 'thunder and lightning', full of Bliss and heavenly sounds. For, saith the Great Law:

> "In order to become the knower of ALL-SELF thou hast first of Self to be the knower. To reach the knowledge of

> that Self, thou hast to give up Self to Non-Self, Being to Non-Being, and then thou canst repose between the wings of the GREAT BIRD. Aye, sweet is rest between the wings of that which is not born, nor dies, but is the AUM throughout eternal ages."[62]

3. RASĀNANDA-YOGA-SAMĀDHI

10. Drawing in the air slowly (perform the Bhrāmarī-kumbhaka) and expire more and more slowly (as if stopping to listen); a rumbling sound like that of a buzzing bee will arise.
11. Place the Manas (consciousness) in the centre of this inner humming. This leads to Samādhi and untold Bliss; and the experience of 'Soham' (He am I) arises.

Rasānanda-yoga-samādhi has for sole 'support' the Sound element (Anāhata-śabda). Some blissful sounds, in increasing degrees of sweetness, arise from the immaculate Void of the Heart (see commentary on V, 82). With consciousness fully absorbed in the centre of this inner humming—the reverberating Word of Life—the Yogin waits, expectant yet serene, without desire, until the sound current carries him upwards (inwards) to the gates of Liberation and untold Bliss. For,

> "That which is the sound 'AUM' O Satyakāma, is verily the higher and the lower Brahman. Therefore, with this support alone does the wise man reach the one or the other."[63]

or, as the Maitrī Upaniṣad fully describes it:

> "There are, verily, two Brahmans to be meditated upon, sound and non-sound. By sound alone is the non-sound revealed. Now here the sound is AUM. Moving upward by it one comes to ascend in the non-sound. So (one says) this is the way, this is immortality, this is complete union and also tranquillity. And now as the spider moves upward by the thread, obtains free space, thus assuredly, indeed, the meditator moving upward by the syllable AUM

obtains independence! Other expounders of the Sound (as Brahman) think otherwise. By closing the ears with the thumbs, they hear the sound of the space within the heart. There is the sevenfold comparison of it; like rivers, a bell, a brass vessel, a wheel, the croaking of frogs, rain, as when one speaks in a still place. Having passed beyond this variously characterised (sounds), they disappear (become merged) in the Supreme, the non-sound, the unmanifest Brahman. There they are characterized and indistinguishable like the various juices that have reached the condition of honey. For thus has it been said, 'There are two Brahmans to be known, the Sound Brahman and what is higher. Those who know the Sound Brahman get to the higher Brahman'."[64]

4. LAYA-SIDDHI-YOGA-SAMĀDHI

12. Performing the Yoni-mudrā, imagine yourself united to Śakti, and so, enjoy the Bliss of union with Paramātman (The Ultimate Reality).
13. By the realization 'I am Brahman', you will become full of Bliss and will reach Advaita-samādhi (One without a second).

It is said that success in Yoni-mudrā paves the way to perfect concentration and mastery of the elements (Tattvas). United to Śakti, the Yogin's consciousness aspires to the highest. Technically speaking—in terms of the Mudrā-System—this Laya-siddhi-yoga-samādhi deals with the inner and subtle processes which occur from Mūlādhāra to Viśuddha-cakra, and, eventually, leads to union with Paramātman or the Ultimate Reality. It is the sphere of Kuṇḍalinī proper, the stage of Laya-yoga, and has nothing to do with the misguided sexual practices indulged in by some schools of Tāntric Yoga and other misguided individuals. He who, lacking in purity, chooses to meddle with this Kuṇḍalinī, is literally playing with fire.

5. BHAKTI-YOGA-SAMĀDHI

14. Imagine within your heart your special Deity in her peculiar

Ishta Devata
in ♡ Manasa Puja

form. Such devotional meditation will provide you with the sweetest ecstasy.

15. In blissful excitement, shedding tears of joy, one becomes entranced. This leads to Samādhi, and the mind becomes peaceful and illumined (Manonmanī).

Bhakti-yoga has for 'support' both the Gross and the Light elements, and it is easy to recognize in it, for example, the Yoga of the Christian Faith, with its emphasis on the devotional side of life, where the Church is the guru and Christ the Iṣṭa-devatā, and the almost exclusive cultivation of the Heart cakra. This is not to say that the higher aspects of Yoga are not present in Christian Mysticism, as a simple examination of the work of masters of the spiritual life, such as St. John of the Cross and St. Teresa of Avila clearly indicates, as shown in the following passages:

> "The Heavenly Father has uttered only one word: it is his Son. He says it eternally and in an Eternal Silence. It is in the Silence of the soul that it makes itself heard."[65]

and,

> "As I write this, the noises in my head are so loud that I am beginning to wonder what is going on in it. As I said at the outset, they have been making it almost impossible for me to obey those who commanded me to write. My head sounds just as if it were full of brimming rivers, and then as if all the water in those rivers came suddenly rushing downwards; and a host of little birds seem to be whistling, not in the ears, but in the upper part of the head, where the higher part of the soul is said to be."[66]

Anyone who seriously follows the path of Yoga will come to recognize in the above colourful description certain unmistakable signs normally present in its most highest reaches. Sometimes, communion with the Word can prove to be a very disconcerting experience, as the words of that fine observer, St. Teresa, obviously prove. Such description corresponds very closely to certain stages of Nāda-yoga-samādhi. As it is normally the case in

Bhakti-yoga, the experience must have come to the Spanish saint via the 'citta-vāhā-nāḍī', a subtle mystical link which connects the heart with the brain.

6. RĀJA-YOGA-SAMĀDHI

16. Performing Manomūrcchā-kumbhaka, unite your thinking principle (Manas) with the Self (Ātman). By this union with Paramātman, one reaches Rāja-yoga-samādhi.

We have come now to the natural outcome of Haṭha-yoga: Rāja-yoga-samādhi. This is the King of Yogas and represents the Royal Path. In the same way as the various energies which go to form a personality (with all its various subtle aspects) had to be purified, harmonized, transmuted and reabsorbed into its pristine essence by means of Prāṇāyāma, Pratyāhāra, Dhyāna and the various Samādhis, it is now time for the Mind itself to become absorbed in the Self (Ātman). This is why the Yogin is told to perform Manomūrcchā-(mental) kumbhaka (see also V, 83) the highest, the subtlest Kumbhaka of all-true Prāṇāyāma. For what is Prāṇāyāma? "Literally translated it means the 'death' of vital breath...The Tāntrikas take it literally, as relating to the regulation of the vital, lung breath, whereas the ancient Rāja-yogins understood it as referring to the mental or 'WILL BREATH', which alone leads to the function of the 'THIRD EYE', and the acquisition of the true Rāja-yoga occult powers."[67] Success in this Samādhi confers upon the Yogin the right to enter the practice of the highest Yoga, described by Patañjali as 'citta-vṛtti-nirodhaḥ', for only

> "By controlling and ultimately suppressing the activity of the individual mind is attained knowledge of the Ātman or the individual Spirit in man."[68]

Or, to put it in the words of that priceless gift to theosophical literature, The Voice of the Silence:

> "Silence thy thoughts and fix thy whole attention on thy Master whom yet thou doest not see, but whom thou feelest. Merge into one sense thy senses if thou wouldst be

secure against the foe. Tis by that sense alone which lies concealed within the hollow of thy brain, that the steep path which leadeth to thy Master may be disclosed before thy soul's dim eyes."[69]

Unlike the other Yogas, this Rāja-yoga-samādhi has the Mind itself for sole 'support'. It is the most subtle of all Yogas and so it comes as no surprise to know that it has been misunderstood nearly as often as its companion, Haṭha-yoga; for, extremes do happen to meet each other in the most mysterious ways. It is to the Yogin standing on the threshold of Rāja-yoga that the following mystical words are addressed:

"Thyself and mind, like twins upon a line, the star which is thy goal burns overhead."[70]

Thus referring to the Secret Three, the Mystic Triangle (△) of Rāja-yoga. This is the sphere of Awesome Silence and unimaginable Splendour; of lasting Bliss and Liberation.

SUBLIMITY OF SAMĀDHI-YOGA

17. O Caṇḍa! Thus have I instructed you on Samādhi which leads to liberation. Rāja-yoga-samādhi, Unmanī, Sahajāvasthā, they all mean union with the Self (Ātman).
18. The Omnipresent Viṣṇu is in the water; he is in the earth; he is on the top of a mountain; he is in the midst of volcanic fires and flames. The entire universe is full of Viṣṇu.
19. All living and animate creation that moves on land or air, trees, shrubs, climbers, grass and other plants; oceans and mountain ranges, know these all to be Brahman. See them all in Ātman.
20. The Ātman abiding in the body is Caitanya (Pure Consciousness); One without a second, Eternal, Supreme. Knowing it as separate from the body, one conquers all desires and passions.
21. Thus Samādhi is free from all desires. Without attachment to his own body, to son, wife, friends or riches, let one reach Samādhi.
22. Śiva has revealed many hidden Truths (Tattvas) such as Laya-amṛta, etc; of these, I have given you a brief summary leading to liberation.

23. O Caṇḍa! Thus have I told you about the great Samādhi, difficult of attainment. He who realizes this, ceases to be born.

In the same way as the various Mudrās had to be placed in their proper sequential order, so as to discover their true significance, the various Samādhis also follow a certain natural sequence and cannot be treated arbitrarily; the sequence being as follows: (1) Bhakti-yoga, (2) Rasānanda-yoga, (3) Laya-siddhi-yoga, (4) Dhyāna-yoga, (5) Nāda-yoga, and (6) Rāja-yoga; thus forming an uninterrupted and perfectly integrated whole; it begins with conscious Love and Devotion and ends in super-conscious Bliss and Wisdom. The discerning student will see that there is an almost perfect correspondence between these various Samādhis and the other various elements of Yoga as described in this text, i.e. Mudrās, Prāṇāyāma, Dhyāna When properly understood (the veil being partially cast aside) this little Yoga treatise is found to form a Pure Yoga-System, where the individual parts fit, with extraordinary accuracy, with each other, in perfect union. "Equilibrium is called Yoga."[71] Such is the Yoga of the Gheraṇḍa-saṃhitā, a perfectly harmonious blend of hidden truths, intended by the Lord Śiva to reveal the mysteries of the Self.

EPILOGUE

The sole purpose of this new book on Yoga has been to attempt to dispel some of the misconceptions and errors prevalent in today's presentation of the Sacred Science. In fact, to bring this back to its original purity in whatever measure this may be possible.

It has not been the intention of the author to reveal more than it would have been prudent to reveal. This is why certain key elements are absent from the commentary. But enough has been given to allow the pure seeker after Yoga to come to a sound and healthy understanding of the subject.

No teaching, however, can ever be a perfect substitute for Yoga. And no teacher or guru will ever be a real and perfect substitute for that Inner Guru who, silently and patiently, awaits that blissful moment when the disciple is ready to see the light. That light from the One Master (Mahā-guru) the one unfading golden light of spirit which, from the very first, shines upon the true disciple.

TATTVAMASI

REFERENCES

1. Īśāvāsya Upaniṣad, 9
2. Laghu-yoga-vāsiṣṭha, p. 296, Adyar ed.
3. Bhagavadgītā, IV, 2-3
4. Patañjali-yoga-sūtra, I, 24-27
5. Laghu-yoga-Śrī Śaṅkarācārya, p. 296, Adyar ed.
6. St. John's Gospel, I, 1-5
7. Śiva-sūtra, I, 5
8. 'The Golden Stairs', H.P. Blavatsky
9. Gāyatrī, I. K. Taimni, p. 153
10. St. Matthew's Gospel, XI, 14-15
11. St. John's Gospel, IX, 2
12. The Book of Revelation, III, 12
13. Aparokṣānubhūti of Śrī-śaṅkarācārya, verse 116
14. Haṭha-yoga-pradīpikā, I, 39-41
15. Aparokṣānubhūti, verse 114
16. Haṭha-yoga-pradīpikā, IV, 43
17. Laghu-yoga-vāsiṣṭha, p. 68, Adyar ed.
18. Laghu-yoga-vāsiṣṭha, p. 268, Adyar ed.
19. Śiva-sūtra, III, 5
20. Light on the Path (little essay on 'Karma'), p. 100, M. Collins
21. Śiva-sūtra, III, 6
22. Laghu-yoga-vāsiṣṭha, p. 341, Adyar ed.
23. Wisdom of Solomon (Apocrypha) II, 23
24. Kaṭha Upaniṣad, II, i, 1
25. Patañjali-yoga-sūtra, II, 54-55
26. Aparokṣānubhūti, verse 121
27. Haṭha-yoga-pradīpikā, II, 12
28. Bhagavad-gītā, VIII, 12-13
29. Laghu-yoga-vāsiṣṭha, p. 311, Adyar ed.
30. Bhagavad-gītā, XVII, 8-10
31. Chāndogya Upaniṣad, VIII, iii, 5
32. Aparokṣānubhūti, verses 119-20
33. The Voice of the Silence, I, 2, H.P. Blavatsky
34. The Voice of the Silence, I, 42-49, H.P. Blavatsky
35. Laghu-yoga-vāsiṣṭha, p. 307-8, Adyar ed.
36. Bhagavad-gītā, IV, 29
37. The Lotus Fire, p. 272, G.S. Arundale
38. Patañjali-yoga-sūtra, II, 49-51
39. The Lotus Fire, p. 386, G.S. Arundale
40. Light on the Path, I, 21, Mabel Collins
41. Patañjali-yoga-sūtra, II, 52-53
42. Laghu-yoga-vāsiṣṭha, pp. 338-39, Adyar ed.

43. Aparokṣānubhūti, verse 118
44. Bhagavad-gītā, VI, 35
45. Yogatārāvalī of Śrīśaṅkarācārya
46. Bhagavad-gītā, VI, 19
47. Patañjali-yoga-sūtra, II, 52
48. Patañjali-yoga-sūtra, III, 26
49. St. John's Gospel, III, 13-15
50. The Secret Doctrine, Vol. III, p. 503, H.P. Blavatsky
51. The Book of Revelation, XXI, 24-25
52. The Secret Doctrine, Vol. III, pp. 504-5, H.P. Blavatsky
53. Patañjali-yoga-sūtra, III, 2-3
54. Śiva-sūtra, II, 7
55. The Voice of the Silence, I, 80-81, H.P. Blavatsky
56. The Voice of the Silence, I, 82-83, H.P. Blavatsky
57. The Lotus Fire, p. 149, G.S. Arundale
58. The Book of Revelation, VIII, 1
59. Īśāvāsya Upaniṣad, verse 15
60. Bhagavad-gītā, V, 27-28
61. St. Matthew's Gospel, XXVII, 33
62. The Voice of the Silence, I, 19, H.P. Blavatsky
63. Praśna Upaniṣad, V, 2
64. Maitrī Upaniṣad, VI, 22
65. Complete Works of St. John of the Cross, Maxim 307
66. The Interior Castle, IV Mansions, II, 234, St. Teresa of Avila
67. The Secret Doctrine, Vol. III, 503, H.P. Blavatsky
68. Siva-sūtra, I, 17
69. The Voice of the Silence, I, 72-73, H.P. Blavatsky
70. The Voice of the Silence, I, 88, H.P. Blavatsky
71. Bhagavad-gītā, II, 48

LIST OF SANSKRIT WORKS

AND OTHER SOURCES TO WHICH DIRECT REFERENCE HAS BEEN MADE IN THIS BOOK

Āditya Purāṇa
Aparokṣānubhūti
Ātmabodha
Bhagavad-gītā
Bhāgavata Purāṇa
Brahma-bindu Upaniṣad
Brahma-vidyā Upaniṣad
Chāndogya Upaniṣad
Devībhāgavata
Devīgītā
Dhyāna-bindu Upaniṣad
Garuḍa Purāṇa
Gorakṣa-saṃhitā
Haṃsa Upaniṣad
Hastāmalaka-stotra
Haṭha-yoga-pradīpikā
Īśāvāsya Upaniṣad
Kaṭha Upaniṣad
Kūrma Purāṇa
Laghu-yogavāsiṣṭha
Laws of Manu
Maitrī Upaniṣad
Maṇḍala-brāhmaṇa Upaniṣad
Nāda-bindu Upaniṣad
Patañjali-yoga-sūtra
Prabodhasudhākara
Praśna Upaniṣad
Śiva-saṃhitā
Śiva-sūtra
Skanda Purāṇa
Śrīmadbhāgavata
Śvetāśvatara Upaniṣad
Tejo-bindu Upaniṣad
Triśikhī-brāhmaṇa Upaniṣad
Viṣṇu Purāṇa
Viveka-Cūḍāmaṇi
Yājñavalkya-saṃhitā
Yogabīja Upaniṣad
Yogacintāmaṇi
Yoga-sāra-saṅgraha
Yoga-śikhā Upaniṣad
Yogatārāvalī
Yoga-tattva Upaniṣad

COMPLETE WORKS OF ST. JOHN OF THE CROSS
Gāyatrī, I.K. Taimni
Light on the Path, Mabel Collins
The Gospel according to St. John
The Gospel according to St. Matthew
The Interior Castle, St. Teresa of Avila
The Lotus Fire, George Arundale
The Revelation of St. John the Divine
The Secret Doctrine, H.P. Blavatsky
The Voice of the Silence, H.P. Blavatsky
The Wisdom of Solomon (Apocrypha)

GLOSSARY OF SANSKRIT WORDS

Ādhāra—support.

Ādi—first and highest.

Ādinātha—Lord of the world.

Ādiśvara—primeval Lord, first Creator, Śiva.

Agni-tattva—'fire' as a cosmic element.

Ahaṃkāra—'I' making faculty, Ego, egotism.

Ajapā-mantra—this is the 'wordless' mantra, the unconscious, continuous prayer of all life; the breathing of all living creatures produces a double sound: the inward breath sounds like "So'ham" (Saḥ=He—the Universal Self; 'aham'=am I) and the outward breath sounds like 'Haṃsaḥ' (Aham=I am; Saḥ=He—the Universal Self).

Ājñā-cakra—subtle centre of command situated between the eyebrows, sometimes referred to as 'the Third Eye'.

Ākāśa—Space, the subtlest of the five 'mystic' elements, itself admitting of gradations of subtlety.

Anāhata-cakra—subtle centre corresponding to the cardiac region (Heart cakra).

Anāhata-śabda—eternal sound current; the 'song' of the purified heart of the Yogin; the touch of Grace.

Ānanda—Infinite Bliss.

Ananta—infinite, eternal; symbolized by a snake swallowing its tail.

Apāna—one of the vital airs, ruling the lower abdominal region; the inhaled air.

Ap-tattva—'water' as a cosmic element.

Āsana—posture.

Atiśūnya—the 'middle void', the sphere of influence of the purified Viśuddha (Throat) cakra.

Ātman—Oversoul, Spirit, Brahman, Self.

Aum—the Sacred Word, the Word made Flesh; the Hindu symbol for the Ultimate Reality in manifestation.

Bandha—fetter, lock; interlocking posture of certain organs or parts of the body.

Bhakti—adoration, devotion, mystical love, worship.

Bhūtas—the five elements as stimulators of the senses.

Bhutākāśa—elemental Space; material and astral realms.

Bīja—seed, germ.

Bindu—point, drop.

Brahmā—the Creator, the first deity of the Hindu Trinity (Brahmā, Viṣṇu, Śiva).

Brahman—the Supreme Being; the Spirit of the Universe, God.

Brahmarandhra—top cakra; a subtle 'aperture' in the crown of the head which enables the adept to secure release from the bonds of the material world.

Buddhi—intuition, higher reason, spiritual discrimination, unclouded, pure vision; the seventh Tattva.

Cakra—wheel, circle, plexus; subtle organ in man's invisible anatomy (see Table 1); centre serving as instrument or means of communication and interplay of forces between man's various vehicles of consciousness.

Cakra-bheda—piercing of the cakra.

Celā—disciple.

Cidākāśa—spiritual Space (realm).

Cit—consciousness, the Absolute.

Citta—the mind, comprising all its various faculties, i.e. selection, rejection, analysis, attention, egoism, etc.

Cittākāśa—mental Space (realm).

Citta-vāhā-nāḍī—subtle link in man's invisible anatomy connecting the 'heart' with the 'mind'.

Citta-vṛtti-nirodhaḥ—subsidence of the modifications of the mind; like the waters of a lake suddenly turned profoundly calm.

Deva—a god.

Dhāraṇā—Concentration; total attention, one-pointedness; Patañjali's sixth Yoga stage.

Dhyāna—Meditation; continuous concentration, effortless, like an uninterrupted flow of oil; Patañjali's seventh Yoga stage.

Gāyatrī—well-known Hindu mantra meaning:
"We meditate upon the Divine Light of that ineffable Sun of Spiritual Consciousness which enhances our power of spiritual perception."

Gheraṇḍa—famous Sage, author of the Gheraṇḍa-saṃhitā.

Guṇas—qualities of Prakṛti (Nature) found to be threefold: Rajas (mobility, activity; to use an analogy, the electron) Tamas (inertia, darkness; to use an analogy, the neutron) and Sattva (equilibrium, balance, harmony, rhythm; to use an analogy, the proton).

Guru—Teacher, Spiritual Guide.

Ha—first syllable of the word Haṭha, meaning, among other things, 'Sun'; symbol of Śakti or Divine Power.

Haṃsa—a swan, symbol of spiritual discernment.

Haṃsaḥ—'I am He'; the Universal Self; it constitutes one half of the Ajapā-mantra.

Haṭha—force, forcibly; with rigorous effort. Also, thorough and effortless union of Ha (Sun) and Ṭha (Moon).

Iḍā—a nāḍī or channel of subtle energy also called Candra-nāḍī, conveying 'lunar' energy.

Iṣṭa-devatā—chosen deity.

Īśvara—the Supreme Being, God.

Jāgrat—ordinary state of awareness (waking state) on any place of being.

Japa—repetitive prayer.

Jīvātman—the individual soul.

Jñāna—Divine Wisdom.

Kaivalya—Independence, Isolation, Self-realization, Perfect Liberation, Total Self-awareness.

Karma—action and reaction.

Kevala—absolute, total, perfect, pure.

Kevala-kumbhaka—perfect subsidence of the Breath, generally understood as 'retention'.

Khecarī—to move in the sky (Space).

Kriyā—practice.

Kuṇḍalinī-śakti—pristine, creative energy, said to be coiled up like a serpent, slumbering in the deepest recesses of man's subtle anatomy. It is said to reside in the lowest cakra (Mūlādhāra) the root and support of individual manifestation; the Serpent Fire. Some authorities place it in the third cakra.

Laya—dissolution, subsidence; total mental absorption in a higher state of consciousness.

Laya-yoga—union with the Divine by means of intense and pure devotion; ecstatic rapture; communion with the Sacred Word (nāda).

Mahākāśa—the subtlest Space.

Mahāśūnya—the 'Great Void'; the sphere of influence of the purified Ājñā-cakra.

Manas—the 'lower' mind with its basic functions of comparison, rejection, acceptance, analysis, etc.

Maṇipūra-cakra—subtle centre corresponding to the solar plexus or abdominal 'brain'.

Mantra—a sacred word or prayer; incantation.

Mātṛkā-cakra—combination of 'spiritual' sounds operating through a central and common mechanism of inner perception; access to such mechanism is only possible to a realized individual.

Māyā—Illusion.

Mudrā—a seal; a sealing posture; secret; the core of tantric Yoga.

Mukti—liberation, perfect Self-realization.

Mūlādhāra-cakra—subtle centre corresponding to the coccygeal region (Root cakra).

Nāda—inner mystical sound; it has no beginning and no end; it is a subtle, eternal, infinite, reverberating vibration experienced in the higher reaches of Laya-yoga; integrated 'Sound', the matrix of all vibrations.

Nāḍī—subtle channel of energy found in the human body; there exist innumerable nāḍīs but three of these are of special importance to the Yogin: Iḍā (left nostril) Piṅgalā (right nostril) and Suṣumnā (inner core of spinal column).

Nirodha—restrain, control, inhibition; subsidence.

Nirvāṇa—Samādhi, Kaivalya.

Om—same as Aum; the Sacred Word, the Word of Life; the Word no human lips on earth, no mortal mind is ever pure enough to pronounce. The essence of the Vedas, representing the Supreme Truth, the Ultimate Reality.

Paramātman—Supreme Spirit.

Patañjali-yoga-sūtra—the classical Raja-yoga 'textbook' used by a great many practitioners of the higher aspects of Yoga.

Piṅgalā—a nāḍī or channel of subtle energy, also called sūrya-nāḍī, conveying 'solar' energy.

Prakṛti—Nature, Matter; the opposite or rather, complement of Spirit which manifests by means of three basic qualities or Guṇas, i.e. Rajas, Tamas and Sattva.

Pralaya—cosmic state of latency, dissolution, 'suspended animation' of a Universe.

Prāṇa—breath, vitality, life, wind; subtle psychic energy; total energy; the exhaled air.

Praṇava—another word for Om or Aum.

Prāṇāyāma—rhythmic control of the breath (prāṇa); subtle 'expansion' of the breath inwards and outwards. This is a secret.

Pratyāhāra—withdrawal of the mind from the sense-organs and sensual objects.

Pṛthivī—one of the five elements referred to as 'Earth'.

Pūraka—inspiration.

Purāṇas—a class of Hindu scriptures.

Puruṣa—the individual spirit.

Rāja-yoga—The royal road in Yoga. Patañjali's eightfold Yoga; union with the Supreme by means of complete mind control and mastery of the inner nature; regeneration and 'birth' of the Spiritual Mind.

Rajas—one of the three Guṇas or modes of Prakṛti (Nature) meaning activity, mobility, restlessness.

Recaka—expiration.

Śabda—mystical sound (Word).

Sādhaka—spiritual aspirant.

Sādhana—spiritual discipline; self-culture; training.

Sahasrāra-cakra—the thousand-petalled lotus in the top of the head.

Śakti—from one point of view, there are two principles in the Universe, Śiva (consciousness) and Śakti (Energy or Power). Śakti is the totality of Power, be this latent or manifest.

Samādhi—state of total absorption, when the observer (thinker, knower) and the observed (thought, thing) are one.

Samāna—one of the vital airs; it aids the power of digestion.

Śāmbhavī—belonging to Śambhu or Śiva.

Saṃsāra—wheel of births and deaths.

Śāstras—certain Hindu scriptures.

Saccidānanda—Being—Consciousness—Bliss; the crown of Self-realization; man's true inner nature.

Sattva—one of the three Guṇas of Prakṛti (Nature) symbolising harmony, rhythm.

Siddha—perfected human being; self-realized individual.

Siddhi—accomplishment, perfection, power.

Śiva—third god of the Hindu Trinity; the Destroyer; also the supreme 'patron' of Yogins.

Soham—'He am I'; one part of the Ajapā-mantra.

Sthūla—gross, material.

Sūkṣma—subtle.

Śūnya—the Void; the sphere of influence of the purified Anāhata-cakra.

Suṣumnā—mystical 'mechanism' of Self-realization; the main subtle channel corresponding to the inner 'portion' of the spinal column; it constitutes the path of Liberation—the secret path, the pathway of Kuṇḍalinī-śakti or pristine spiritual energy.

Suṣupti—dreamless state.

Svādhiṣṭhāna-cakra—subtle centre corresponding to the sacral plexus.

Svapna—dreaming state.

Tamas—darkness, ignorance; one of the three Guṇas or qualities of Prakṛti (Nature).

Tattva—primordial, original principle; primary 'substance'.

Tattva-jñāna—knowledge (experience) of the essential Principle: the Truth; knowing which, all else is known.

Tattvamasi—'That Thou art'; the supreme realization that man is a spiritual being; the Divine abides within him; it is, in fact, his very nature. The only way to discover this simple truth is by means of intense Self-realization.

Tejas—brilliance, fire; one of the five elements, related to light.

Ṭha—second syllable of the word Haṭha, meaning, among other things, 'moon'.

Trāṭaka—fixed, rigid gaze; secret Yoga practice to steady the mind.

Udāna—one of the vital airs, corresponding to the thoracic region and controlling the intake of food and air.

Upādhi—vehicle of consciousness, sheath.

Vasiṣṭha—a most celebrated Sage; a true Jñānin (Wise Man) propounder of the most excellent form of Vedāntic teaching.

Vāyu—one of the five elements called 'Air'.

Vedānta—the latter part of the Vedas; the crown of the Hindu spiritual message of Liberation and Enlightenment.

Viṣṇu—the Preserver; the second deity of the Hindu Trinity.

Viśuddha-cakra—subtle centre corresponding to the laryngeal plexus (Throat cakra).

Vṛtti—modification, transformation.

Vyāna—one of the vital airs; it permeates the whole body.

घेरण्डसंहिता

प्रथमोपदेशः ।

आदीश्वराय प्रणमामि तस्मै येनोपदिष्टा हठयोगविद्या ।
विराजते प्रोन्नतराजयोगमारोढुमिच्छोरधिरोहिणीव ।।

घटस्थयोगकथनम् ।

एकदा चण्डकापालिर्गत्वा घेरण्डकुट्टिरम् ।
प्रणम्य विनयाद् भक्त्या घेरण्डं परिपृच्छति ।।१।।

श्रीचण्डकापालिरुवाच—

घटस्थयोगं योगेश तत्त्वज्ञानस्य कारणम् ।
इदानीं श्रोतुमिच्छामि योगेश्वर वद प्रभो ।।२।।

घेरण्ड उवाच—

साधु साधु महाबाहो यन्मां त्वं परिपृच्छसि ।
कथयामि हि ते वत्स सावधानोऽवधारय ।।३।।

नास्ति मायासमः पाशो नास्ति योगात्परं बलम् ।
नास्ति ज्ञानात्परो बन्धुर्नाहंकारात्परो रिपुः ।।४।।

अभ्यासात्कादिवर्णानां यथा शास्त्राणि बोधयेत् ।
तथा योगं समासाद्य तत्त्वज्ञानं च लभ्यते ।।५।।

सुकृतैर्दुष्कृतैः कार्यैर्जायते प्राणिनां घटः ।
घटादुत्पद्यते कर्म घटीयन्त्रं यथा भ्रमेत् ।।६।।

ऊर्ध्वाधो भ्रमते यद्वद्घटीयन्त्रं गवां वशात् ।
तद्वत्कर्मवशाज्जीवो भ्रमते जन्ममृत्युभिः ।।७।।

आमकुम्भ इवाम्भःस्थो जीर्यमाणः सदा घटः ।
योगानलेन संदह्य घटशुद्धिं समाचरेत् ।।८।।

अथ सप्तसाधनम्

शोधनं दृढता चैव स्थैर्यं धैर्यं च लाघवम् ।
प्रत्यक्षं च निर्लिप्तं च घटस्य सप्तसाधनम् ।।९।।

अथ सप्तसाधनलक्षणम् ।

षट्कर्मणा शोधनं च आसनेन भवेद् दृढम् ।
मुद्रया स्थिरता चैव प्रत्याहारेण धीरता ॥१०॥

प्राणायामाल्लाघवं च ध्यानात्प्रत्यक्षमात्मनः ।
समाधिना निर्लिप्तं च मुक्तिरेव न संशयः ॥११॥

अथ शोधनम् ।

धौतिर्वस्तिस्तथा नेतिर्लौलिकी त्राटकं तथा ।
कपालभातिश्चैतानि षट्कर्माणि समाचरेत् ॥१२॥

अथ धौतिः ।

अन्तर्धौतिर्दन्तधौतिर्हृद्धौतिर्मूलशोधनम् ।
धौतिं चतुर्विधां कृत्वा घटं कुर्वन्तु निर्मलम् ॥१३॥

अथ अन्तर्धौतिः ।

वातसारं वारिसारं वह्निसारं बहिष्कृतम् ।
घटस्य निर्मलार्थाय ह्यन्तर्धौतिश्चतुर्विधा ॥१४॥

अथ वातसारः ।

काकचञ्चूवदास्येन पिबेद्वायुं शनैः शनैः ।
चालयेदुदरं पश्चाद्वर्त्मना रेचयेच्छनैः ॥१५॥

वातसारं परं गोप्यं देहनिर्मलकारणम् ।
सर्वरोगक्षयकरं देहानलविवर्धकम् ॥१६॥

अथ वारिसारः ।

आकण्ठं पूरयेद्वारि वक्त्रेण च पिबेच्छनैः ।
चालयेदुदरेणैव चोदराद्रेचयेदधः ॥१७॥

वारिसारं परं गोप्यं देहनिर्मलकारकम् ।
साधयेत्तत्प्रयत्नेन देवदेहं प्रपद्यते ॥१८॥

वारिसारं परां धौतिं साधयेद्यः प्रयत्नतः ।
मलदेहं शोधयित्वा देवदेहं प्रपद्यते ॥१९॥

अथ अग्निसारः ।

नाभिग्रन्थिं मेरुपृष्ठे शतवारं च कारयेत् ।
अग्निसार इयं धौतिर्योगिनां योगसिद्धिदा ।
उदर्यमामयं त्यक्त्वा जाठराग्निं विवर्धयेत् ॥२०॥

एषा धौति: परा गोप्या देवानामपि दुर्लभा ।
केवलं धौतिमात्रेण देवदेहो भवेद् ध्रुवम् ॥२१॥

अथ बहिष्कृतधौति: ।

काकीमुद्रां साधयित्वा पूरयेद्बुदुरं मरुत् ।
धारयेदर्धयामं तु चालयेदर्धवर्त्मना ।
एषा धौति: परा गोप्या न प्रकाश्या कदाचन ॥२२॥

अथ प्रक्षालनम् ।

नाभिदघ्ने जले स्थित्वा शक्तिनाडीं विसर्जयेत् ।
कराभ्यां क्षालयेन्नाडीं यावन्मलविसर्जनम् ।
तावत्प्रक्षाल्य नाडीं च उदरे वेशयेत्पुन: ॥२३॥

इदं प्रक्षालनं गोप्यं देवानामपि दुर्लभम् ।
केवलं धौतिमात्रेण देवदेहो भवेद् ध्रुवम् ॥२४॥

अथ बहिष्कृतधौतिप्रयोग: ।

यामार्धं धारणां शक्ति न यावत्साधयेन्नर: ।
बहिष्कृतं महद्धौतिस्तावच्चैव न जायते ॥२५॥

अथ दन्तधौति: ।

दन्तमूलं जिह्वामूलं रन्ध्रं कर्णयुगस्य च ।
कपालरन्ध्रं पञ्चैते दन्तधौति प्रचक्षते ॥२६॥

अथ दन्तमूलधौति: ।

खादिरेण रसेनाथ शुद्धिमृत्तिकया तथा ।
मार्जयेद्दन्तमूलं च यावत्किल्विषमाहरेत् ॥२७॥

दन्तमूलं परा धौतिर्योगिनां योगसाधने ।
नित्यं कुर्यात्प्रभाते च दन्तरक्षां च योगवित् ।
दन्तमूलं धावनादिकार्येषु योगिनां मतम् ॥२८॥

अथ जिह्वाशोधनम् ।

अथात: संप्रवक्ष्यामि जिह्वाशोधनकारणम् ।
जरामरणरोगादीन्नाशयेद्दीर्घलम्बिका ॥२९॥

अथ जिह्वामूलधौतिप्रयोग: ।

तर्जनीमध्यमानामाख्याङ्गुलित्रययोगत: ।
वेशयेद् गलमध्ये तु मार्जयेल्लम्बिकामलम् ।
शनै: शनैर्मार्जयित्वा कफदोषं निवारयेत् ॥३०॥

मार्जयेन्नवनीतेन दोहयेच्च पुनः पुनः ।
तदग्रं लौहयन्त्रेण कर्षयित्वा शनैः शनैः ॥३१॥
नित्यं कुर्यात्प्रयत्नेन रवेरुदयकेऽस्तके ।
एवं कृते च नित्यं सा लम्बिका दीर्घतां व्रजेत् ॥३२॥

अथ कर्णधौतिप्रयोगः ।

तर्जन्यनामिकायोगान्मार्जयेत्कर्णरन्ध्रयोः ।
नित्यमभ्यासयोगेन नादान्तरं प्रकाशयेत् ॥३३॥

अथ कपालरन्ध्रप्रयोगः ।

वृद्धाङ्गुष्ठेन दक्षेण मार्जयेद्भालरन्ध्रकम् ।
एवमभ्यासयोगेन कफदोषं निवारयेत् ॥३४॥
नाडी निर्मलतां याति दिव्यदृष्टिः प्रजायते ।
निद्रान्ते भोजनान्ते च दिनान्ते च दिने दिने ॥३५॥

अथ हृद्धौतिः ।

हृद्धौतिं त्रिविधां कुर्याद्दण्डवमनवाससा ॥३६॥
रम्भादण्डं हरिद्दण्डं वेत्रदण्डं तथैव च ।
हृन्मध्ये चालयित्वा तु पुनः प्रत्याहरेच्छनैः ॥३७॥
कफं पित्तं तथा क्लेदं रेचयेदूर्ध्ववर्त्मना ।
दण्डधौतिविधानेन हृद्रोगं नाशयेद् ध्रुवम् ॥३८॥

अथ वमनधौतिः ।

भोजनान्ते पिबेद्वारि चाकण्ठं पूरितं सुधीः ।
ऊर्ध्वां दृष्टिं क्षणं कृत्वा तज्जलं वमयेत्पुनः ।
नित्यमभ्यासयोगेन कफपित्तं निवारयेत् ॥३९॥

अथ वासोधौतिः ।

चतुरङ्गुलविस्तारं सूक्ष्मवस्त्रं शनैर्ग्रसेत् ।
पुनः प्रत्याहरेदेतत्प्रोच्यते धौतिकर्मकम् ॥४०॥
गुल्मज्वरप्लीहाकुष्ठकफपित्तं विनश्यति ।
आरोग्यं बलपुष्टिश्च भवेत्तस्य दिने दिने ॥४१॥

अथ मूलशोधनम् ।

अपानक्रूरता तावद्यावन्मूलं न शोधयेत् ।
तस्मात्सर्वप्रयत्नेन मूलशोधनमाचरेत् ॥४२॥
पित्तमूलस्य दण्डेन मध्यमाङ्गुलिनाऽपि वा ।
यत्नेन क्षालयेद् गुह्यं वारिणा च पुनः पुनः ॥४३॥

वारयेत्कोष्ठकाठिन्यमामजीर्णं निवारयेत् ।
कारणं कान्तिपुष्ट्योश्च वह्निमण्डलदीपनम् ।।४४।।

अथ वस्तिप्रकरणम् ।

जलवस्तिः शुष्कवस्तिर्वस्तिः स्याद् द्विविधा स्मृता ।
जलवस्तिं जले कुर्याच्छुष्कवस्तिं सदा क्षितौ ।।४५।।

अथ जलवस्तिः ।

नाभिदघ्ने जले पायुं न्यस्तवानुत्कटासनम् ।
आकुञ्चनं प्रसारं च जलवस्तिं समाचरेत् ।।४६।।

प्रमेहं च उदावर्तं क्रूरवायुं निवारयेत् ।
भवेत्स्वच्छन्ददेहश्च कामदेवसमो भवेत् ।।४७।।

अथ स्थलवस्तिः ।

पश्चिमोत्तानतो वस्तिं चालयित्वा शनैरधः ।
अश्विनीमुद्रया पायुमाकुञ्चयेत् प्रसारयेत् ।।४८।।

एवमभ्यासयोगेन कोष्ठदोषो न विद्यते ।
विवर्धयेज्जाठराग्निमामवातं विनाशयेत् ।।४९।।

अथ नेतियोगः ।

वितस्तिमानं सूक्ष्मसूत्रं नासानाले प्रवेशयेत् ।
मुखान्निर्गमयेत्पश्चात् प्रोच्यते नेतिकर्मकम् ।।५०।।

साधनान्नेतिकार्यस्य खेचरीसिद्धिमाप्नुयात् ।
कफदोषा विनश्यन्ति दिव्यदृष्टिः प्रजायते ।।५१।।

अथ लौलिकीयोगः ।

अमन्दवेगेन तुन्दं भ्रामयेत्पार्श्वयोर्द्वयोः ।
सर्वरोगान्निहन्तीह देहानलविवर्धनम् ।।५२।।

अथ त्राटकम् ।

निमेषोन्मेषकं त्यक्त्वा सूक्ष्मलक्ष्यं निरीक्षयेत् ।
पतन्ति यावदश्रूणि त्राटकं प्रोच्यते बुधैः ।।५३।।

एवमभ्यासयोगेन शांभवी जायते ध्रुवम् ।
नेत्ररोगा विनश्यन्ति दिव्यदृष्टिः प्रजायते ।।५४।।

अथ कपालभातिः ।

वामक्रमेण व्युत्क्रमेण शीत्क्रमेण विशेषतः ।
भालभातिं त्रिधा कुर्यात्कफदोषं निवारयेत् ।।५५।।

अथ वामक्रमकपालभातिः ।

इडया पूरयेद्वायं रेचयेत्पिङ्गलया पुनः ।
पिङ्गलया पूरयित्वा पुनश्चन्द्रेण रेचयेत् ।।५६।।

पूरकं रेचकं कृत्वा वेगेन न तु चालयेत् ।
एवमभ्यासयोगेन कफदोषं निवारयेत् ।।५७।।

अथ व्युत्क्रमकपालभातिः ।

नासाभ्यां जलमाकृष्य पुनर्वक्त्रेण रेचयेत् ।
पायं पायं व्युत्क्रमेण श्लेष्मदोषं निवारयेत् ।।५८।।

अथ शीत्क्रमकपालभातिः ।

शीत्कृत्य पीत्वा वक्त्रेण नासानालैर्विरेचयेत् ।
एवमभ्यासयोगेन कामदेवसमो भवेत् ।।५९।।

न जायते वार्द्धकं च ज्वरो नैव प्रजायते ।
भवेत्स्वच्छन्ददेहश्च कफदोषं निवारयेत् ।।६०।।

इति श्रीघेरण्डसंहितायां घेरण्डचण्डसंवादे षट्कर्मसाधनं
नाम प्रथमोपदेशः समाप्तः ।

द्वितीयोपदेशः ।

अथ आसनानि ।

घेरण्ड उवाच—

आसनानि समस्तानि यावन्तो जीवजन्तवः ।
चतुरशीतिलक्षाणि शिवेन कथितानि च ।।१।।

तेषां मध्ये विशिष्टानि षोडशोनं शतं कृतम् ।
तेषां मध्ये मर्त्यलोके द्वात्रिंशदासनं शुभम् ।।२।।

अथ आसनानां भेदाः ।

सिद्धं पद्मं तथा भद्रं मुक्तं वज्रं च स्वस्तिकम् ।
सिंहं च गोमुखं वीरं धनुरासनमेव च ।।३।।

मृतं गुप्तं तथा मात्स्यं मत्स्येन्द्रासनमेव च ।
गोरक्षं पश्चिमोत्तानमुत्कटं संकटं तथा ।।४।।

मयूरं कुक्कुटं कूर्मं तथा चोत्तानकूर्मकम् ।
उत्तानमण्डुकं वृक्षं मण्डुकं गरुडं वृषम् ।।५।।

शलभं मकरं चोष्ट्रं भुजङ्गं योगमासनम् ।
द्वात्रिंशदासनानां तु मर्त्यलोके हि सिद्धिदा ॥६॥

अथ आसनानां प्रयोगाः ।

अथ सिद्धासनम् ।

योनिस्थानकमङ्घ्रिमूलघटितं संपीड्य गुल्फेतरं
मेढ्रोपर्यथ संनिधाय चिबुकं कृत्वा हृदि स्थापितम् ।
स्थाणुः संयमितेन्द्रियोऽचलदृशा पश्यन्भ्रुवोरन्तरं
ह्येतन्मोक्षकवाटभेदनकरं सिद्धासनं प्रोच्यते ॥७॥

अथ पद्मासनम् ।

वामोरूपरि दक्षिणं हि चरणं संस्थाप्य वामं तथा
दक्षोरूपरि पश्चिमेन विधिना कृत्वा कराभ्यां दृढम् ।
अङ्गुष्ठौ हृदये निधाय चिबुकं नासाग्रमालोकये-
त्सर्वव्याधिविनाशनक्षममिदं पद्मासनं प्रोच्यते ॥८॥

अथ भद्रासनम् ।

गुल्फौ च वृषणस्याधो व्युत्क्रमेण समाहितः ।
पादाङ्गुष्ठौ कराभ्यां च धृत्वा वै पृष्ठदेशतः ॥९॥
जालन्धरं समासाद्य नासाग्रमवलोकयेत् ।
भद्रासनं भवेदेतत्सर्वव्याधिविनाशकम् ॥१०॥

अथ मुक्तासनम् ।

पायुमूले वामगुल्फं दक्षगुल्फं तथोपरि ।
समकायशिरोग्रीवं मुक्तासनं तु सिद्धिदम् ॥११॥

अथ वज्रासनम् ।

जङ्घाभ्यां वज्रवत्कृत्वा गुदपार्श्वे पदावुभौ ।
वज्रासनं भवेदेतद्योगिनां सिद्धिदायकम् ॥१२॥

अथ स्वस्तिकासनम् ।

जानूर्वोरन्तरे कृत्वा योगी पादतले उभे ।
ऋजुकायः समासीत स्वस्तिकं तत्प्रचक्षते ॥१३॥

अथ सिंहासनम् ।

गुल्फौ च वृषणस्याधो व्युत्क्रमेणोर्ध्वतां गतौ ।
चितियुग्मं भूमिसंस्थं हस्तौ कृत्वा च जानुनोः ॥१४॥

व्यात्तवक्त्रो जलन्ध्रेण नासाग्रमवलोकयेत् ।
सिंहासनं भवेदेतत्सर्वव्याधिविनाशकम् ॥१५॥

अथ गोमुखासनम् ।

पादौ च भूमौ संस्थाप्य पृष्ठपार्श्वे निवेशयेत् ।
स्थिरं कायं समासाद्य गोमुखं गोमुखाकृति ॥१६॥

अथ वीरासनम् ।

एकं पादमथैकस्मिन्विन्यसेदूरुसंस्थितम् ।
इतरस्मिंस्तथा पश्चाद्वीरासनमितीरितम् ॥१७॥

अथ धनुरासनम् ।

प्रसार्य पादौ भुवि दण्डरूपौ करद्वयात्ताङ्गुलिपादयुग्मम् ।
कृत्वा धनुर्वत्परिवर्तिताङ्गं निगद्यते वै धनुरासनं तत् ॥१८॥

अथ मृतासनम् ।

उत्तानं शववद् भूमौ शयनं तु शवासनम् ।
शवासनं श्रमहरं चित्तविश्रान्तिकारणम् ॥१९॥

अथ गुप्तासनम् ।

जानूर्वोरन्तरे पादौ कृत्वा पादौ च गोपयेत् ।
पदोपरि च संस्थाप्य गुदं गुप्तासनं विदुः ॥२०॥

अथ मत्स्यासनम् ।

मुक्तपद्मासनं कृत्वा ह्युत्तानशयनं चरेत् ।
कूर्पराभ्यां शिरो वेष्ट्यं रोगघ्नं मात्स्यमासनम् ॥२१॥

अथ मत्स्येन्द्रासनम् ।

उदरं पश्चिमाभासं कृत्वा तिष्ठत्ययत्नतः ।
नम्रितं वामपादं हि दक्षजानूपरि न्यसेत् ॥२२॥

तत्र याम्यं कूर्परं च वक्त्रं याम्यकरेऽपि च ।
भ्रुवोर्मध्ये गता दृष्टिः पीठं मात्स्येन्द्रमुच्यते ॥२३॥

अथ गोरक्षासनम् ।

जानूर्वोरन्तरे पादावुत्तानौ व्यक्तसंस्थितौ ।
गुल्फौ चाच्छाद्य हस्ताभ्यामुत्तानाभ्यां प्रयत्नतः ॥२४॥

कण्ठसंकोचनं कृत्वा नासाग्रमवलोकयेत् ।
गोरक्षासनमित्याह योगिनां सिद्धिकारणम् ॥२५॥

अथ पश्चिमोत्तानासनम् ।

प्रसार्य पादौ भुवि दण्डरूपौ विन्यस्तभालं चितियुग्ममध्ये ।
यत्नेन पादौ च धृतौ कराभ्यां तत्पश्चिमोत्तानमिहासनं स्यात् ॥२६॥

अथ उत्कटासनम् ।

अङ्गुष्ठाभ्यामवष्टभ्य धरां गुल्फौ च खे गतौ ।
तत्रोपरि गुदं न्यस्य विज्ञेयं तूत्कटासनम् ॥२७॥

अथ संकटासनम् ।

वामपादं चितेर्मूलं विन्यस्य धरणीतले ।
पाददण्डेन याम्येन वेष्टयेद्वामपादकम् ।
जानुयुग्मे करयुगमेतत्संकटमासनम् ॥२८॥

अथ मयूरासनम् ।

पाण्योस्तलाभ्यामवलम्ब्य भूमिं तत्कूर्परस्थापितनाभिपार्श्वम् ।
उच्चासनो दण्डवदुत्थितः खे मायूरमेतत्प्रवदन्ति पीठम् ॥२९॥

बहु कदशनभुक्तं भस्म कुर्यादशेषं
जनयति जठराग्निं जारयेत्कालकूटम् ।
हरति सकलरोगानाशु गुल्मज्वरादीन्भवति
विगतदोषं ह्यासनं श्रीमयूरम् ॥३०॥

अथ कुक्कुटासनम् ।

पद्मासनं समासाद्य जान्वोरन्तरे करौ ।
कूर्पराभ्यां समासीन उच्चस्थः कुक्कुटासनम् ॥३१॥

अथ कूर्मासनम् ।

गुल्फौ च वृषणस्याधो व्युत्क्रमेण समाहितौ ।
ऋजुकायशिरोग्रीवं कूर्मासनमितीरितम् ॥३२॥

अथ उत्तानकूर्मकासनम् ।

कुक्कुटासनबन्धस्थं कराभ्यां धृतकन्धरम् ।
पीठं कूर्मवदुत्तानमेतदुत्तानकूर्मकम् ॥३३॥

अथ मण्डुकासनम् ।

पृष्ठदेशे पादतलावङ्गुष्ठौ द्वौ च संस्पृशेत् ।
जानुयुग्मं पुरस्कृत्य साधयेन्मण्डुकासनम् ॥३४॥

अथ उत्तानमण्डुकासनम् ।

मण्डुकासनमध्यस्थं कूर्पराभ्यां धृतं शिरः ।
एतद् भेकवदुत्तानमेतदुत्तानमण्डुकम् ॥३५॥

अथ वृक्षासनम् ।

वामोरुमूलदेशे च याम्यं पादं निधाय वै ।
तिष्ठेत्तु वृक्षवद्भूमौ वृक्षासनमिदं विदुः ।।३६।।

अथ गरुडासनम् ।

जङ्घोरुभ्यां धरां पीडय स्थिरकायो द्विजानुना ।
जानूपरि करद्वन्द्वं गरुडासनमुच्यते ।।३७।।

अथ वृषासनम् ।

याम्यगुल्फे पायुमूलं वामभागे पदेतरम् ।
विपरीतं स्पृशेद्भूमिं वृषासनमिदं भवेत् ।।३८।।

अथ शलभासनम् ।

अध्यास्य शेते करयुग्मवक्षा आलम्ब्य भूमिं करयोस्तलाभ्याम् ।
पादौ च शून्ये च वितस्ति चोर्ध्वं वदन्ति पीठं शलभं मुनीन्द्राः ।।३९।।

अथ मकरासनम् ।

अध्यास्य शेते हृदयं निधाय भूमौ च पादौ प्रविसार्यमाणौ ।
शिरश्च धृत्वा करदण्डयुग्मे देहाग्निकारं मकरासनं तत् ।।४०।।

अथ उष्ट्रासनम् ।

अध्यास्य शेते पदयुग्मव्यस्तं पृष्ठे निधायापि धृतं कराभ्याम् ।
आकुञ्च्य सम्यग्घ्युदरास्यगाढमौष्ट्रं च पीठं यतयो वदन्ति ।।४१।।

अथ भुजङ्गासनम् ।

अङ्गुष्ठनाभिपर्यन्तमधोभूमौ विनिन्यसेत् ।
धरां करतलाभ्यां धृत्वोर्ध्वशीर्षः फणीव हि ।।४२।।

देहाग्निर्वर्धते नित्यं सर्वरोगविनाशनम् ।
जागर्ति भुजगी देवी भुजङ्गासनसाधनात् ।।४३।।

अथ योगासनम् ।

उत्तानौ चरणौ कृत्वा संस्थाप्योपरि जानुनोः ।
आसनोपरि संस्थाप्य चोत्तानं करयुग्मकम् ।।४४।।

पूरकैर्वायुमाकृष्य नासाग्रमवलोकयेत् ।
योगासनं भवेदेतद्योगिनां योगसाधने ।।४५।।

इति श्रीघेरण्डसंहितायां घेरण्डचण्डसंवादे आसनप्रयोगो नाम
द्वितीयोपदेशः समाप्तः ।

तृतीयोपदेशः ।

अथ मुद्राकथनम् ।

घेरण्ड उवाच—

महामुद्रा नभोमुद्रा उड्डीयानं जलन्धरम् ।
मूलबन्धो महाबन्धो महावेधश्च खेचरी ।।१।।
विपरीतकरी योनिर्वज्रोली शक्तिचालनी ।
ताडागी माण्डुकी मुद्रा शांभवी पञ्चधारणा ।।२।।
अश्विनी पाशिनी काकी मातङ्गी च भुजङ्गिनी ।
पञ्चविंशतिमुद्राश्च सिद्धिदा इह योगिनाम् ।।३।।

अथ मुद्राणां फलकथनम् ।

मुद्राणां पटलं देवि कथितं तव संनिधौ ।
येन विज्ञातमात्रेण सर्वसिद्धिः प्रजायते ।।४।।
गोपनीयं प्रयत्नेन न देयं यस्य कस्यचित् ।
प्रीतिदं योगिनां चैव दुर्लभं मरुतामपि ।।५।।

अथ महामुद्राकथनम् ।

पायुमूलं वामगुल्फे संपीडय दृढयत्नतः ।
याम्यपादं प्रसार्याथ करोपात्तपदाङ्गुलिः ।।६।।
कण्ठसंकोचनं कृत्वा भ्रुवोर्मध्यं निरीक्षयेत् ।
महामुद्राभिधा मुद्रा कथ्यते चैव सूरिभिः ।।७।।

अथ महामुद्राफलकथनम् ।

क्षयकासगुदावर्तप्लीहाजीर्णज्वरं तथा ।
नाशयेत्सर्वरोगांश्च महामुद्रा च साधनात् ।।८।।

अथ नभोमुद्राकथनम् ।

यत्र यत्र स्थितो योगी सर्वकार्येषु सर्वदा ।
ऊर्ध्वजिह्वः स्थिरो भूत्वा धारयेत्पवनं सदा ।
नभोमुद्रा भवेदेषा योगिनां रोगनाशिनी ।।९।।

अथ उड्डीयानबन्धः ।

उदरे पश्चिमं तानं नाभेरूर्ध्वं तु कारयेत् ।
उड्डीनं कुरुते यस्मादविश्रान्तं महाखगः ।
उड्डीयानं त्वसौ बन्धो मृत्युमातङ्गकेसरी ।।१०।।

अथ उड्डीयानबन्धस्य फलकथनम् ।

समग्राद् बन्धनाद्ध्येतदुड्डीयानं विशिष्यते ।
उड्डीयाने समभ्यस्ते मुक्तिः स्वाभाविकी भवेत् ॥११॥

अथ जालन्धरबन्धकथनम् ।

कण्ठसंकोचनं कृत्वा चिबुकं हृदये न्यसेत् ।
जालन्धरे कृते बन्धे षोडशाधारबन्धनम् ।
जालन्धरमहामुद्रा मृत्योश्च क्षयकारिणी ॥१२॥

अथ जालन्धरबन्धस्य फलकथनम् ।

सिद्धो जालन्धरो बन्धो योगिनां सिद्धिदायकः ।
षण्मासमभ्यसेद्यो हि स सिद्धो नात्र संशयः ॥१३॥

अथ मूलबन्धकथनम् ।

पार्ष्णिना वामपादस्य योनिमाकुञ्चयेत्ततः ।
नाभिग्रन्थिं मेरुदण्डे सुधीः संपीड्य यत्नतः ॥१४॥
मेढ्रं दक्षिणगुल्फे तु दृढबन्धं समाचरेत् ।
जराविनाशिनी मुद्रा मूलबन्धो निगद्यते ॥१५॥

अथ मूलबन्धस्य फलकथनम् ।

संसारसागरं तर्तुमभिलष्यति यः पुमान् ।
सुगुप्तो विरले भूत्वा मुद्रामेतां समभ्यसेत् ॥१६॥
अभ्यासाद् बन्धनस्यास्य मरुत्सिद्धिर्भवेद् ध्रुवम् ।
साधयेद् यत्नतस्तर्हि मौनी तु विजितालसः ॥१७॥

अथ महाबन्धकथनम् ।

वामपादस्य गुल्फेन पायुमूलं निरोधयेत् ।
दक्षपादेन तद् गुल्फं सुधीः संपीड्य यत्नतः ॥१८॥
शनकैश्चालयेत्पार्ष्णि योनिमाकुञ्चयेच्छनैः ।
जालन्धरे धरेत्प्राणं महाबन्धो निगद्यते ॥१९॥

अथमहाबन्धस्य फलकथनम् ।

महाबन्धः परो बन्धो जरामरणनाशनः ।
प्रसादादस्य बन्धस्य साधयेत्सर्ववाञ्छितम् ॥२०॥

अथ महावेधकथनम् ।

रूपयौवनलावण्यं नारीणां पुरुषं विना ।
मूलबन्धमहाबन्धौ महावेधं विना तथा ॥२१॥

महाबन्धं समासाद्य चरेदुड्डानकुम्भकम् ।
महावेधः समाख्यातो योगिनां सिद्धिदायकः ॥२२॥

अथ महावेधस्य फलकथनम् ।

महाबन्धमूलबन्धौ महावेधसमन्वितौ ।
प्रत्यहं कुरुते यस्तु स योगी योगवित्तमः ॥२३॥

न मृत्युतो भयं तस्य न जरा तस्य विद्यते ।
गोपनीयः प्रयत्नेन वेधोऽयं योगिपुंगवैः ॥२४॥

अथ खेचरीमुद्राकथनम् ।

जिह्वाधो नाडीं संछिन्नां रसनां चालयेत्सदा ।
दोहयेन्नवनीतेन लौहयन्त्रेण कर्षयेत् ॥२५॥

एवं नित्यं समभ्यासाल्लम्बिका दीर्घतां व्रजेत् ।
यावद् गच्छेद् भ्रुवोर्मध्ये तदाऽऽगच्छति खेचरी ॥२६॥

रसनां तालुमध्ये तु शनैः शनैः प्रवेशयेत् ।
कपालकुहरे जिह्वा प्रविष्टा विपरीतगा ।
भ्रुवोर्मध्ये गता दृष्टिर्मुद्रा भवति खेचरी ॥२७॥

अथ खेचरीमुद्रायाः फलकथनम् ।

न च मूर्च्छा क्षुधा तृष्णा नैवालस्यं प्रजायते ।
न च रोगो जरा मृत्युर्देवदेहः स जायते ॥२८॥

नाग्निना दह्यते गात्रं न शोषयति मारुतः ।
न देहं क्लेदयन्त्यापो दशेन्न च भुजङ्गमः ॥२९॥

लावण्यं च भवेद् गात्रे समाधिर्जायते ध्रुवम् ।
कपालवक्त्रसंयोगे रसना रसमाप्नुयात् ॥३०॥

नानारससमुद्भूतमानन्दं च दिने दिने ।
आदौ तु लवणं क्षारं ततस्तिक्तकषायकम् ॥३१॥

नवनीतं घृतं क्षीरं दधितक्रमधूनि च
द्राक्षारसं च पीयूषं जायते रसनोदकम् ॥३२॥

अथ विपरीतकरणीमुद्राकथनम् ।

नाभिमूले वसेत्सूर्यस्तालुमूले च चन्द्रमाः ।
अमृतं ग्रसते सूर्यस्ततो मृत्युवशो नरः ॥३३॥

उर्ध्वे च योजयेत्सूर्यं चन्द्रं चाप्यध आनयेत् ।
विपरीतकरी मुद्रा सर्वतन्त्रेषु गोपिता ॥३४॥

भूमौ शिरश्च संस्थाप्य करयुग्मं समाहितः ।
उर्ध्वपादः स्थिरो भूत्वा विपरीतकरी मता ।।३५।।

अथ विपरीतकरणीमुद्रायाः फलकथनम् ।

मुद्रां च साधयेन्नित्यं जरां मृत्युं च नाशयेत् ।
स सिद्धः सर्वलोकेषु प्रलयेऽपि न सीदति ।।३६।।

अथ योनिमुद्राकथनम् ।

सिद्धासनं समासाद्य कर्णचक्षुर्नसामुखम् ।
अङ्गुष्ठतर्जनीमध्यानामाद्यैः पिदधीत वै ।।३७।।

प्राणमाकृष्य काकीभिरपाने योजयेत्ततः ।
षट् चक्राणि क्रमाद्ध्यात्वा हुं हंसमनुना सुधीः ।।३८।।

चैतन्यमानयेद्देवी निद्रिता या भुजङ्गिनी ।
जीवेन सहितां शक्तिं समुत्थाप्य कराम्बुजे ।।३९।।

स्वयं शक्तिमयो भूत्वा परं शिवेन संगमम् ।
नानासुखं विहारं च चिन्तयेत्परमं सुखम् ।।४०।।

शिवशक्तिसमायोगादेकान्तं भुवि भावयेत् ।
आनन्दमानसो भूत्वा चाहं ब्रह्मेति संभवेत् ।।४१।।

योनिमुद्रा परा गोप्या देवानामपि दुर्लभा ।
सकृत्तु लब्धसंसिद्धिः समाधिस्थः स एव हि ।।४२।।

अथ योनिमुद्राफलकथनम् ।

ब्रह्महा भ्रूणहा चैव सुरापो गुरुतल्पगः ।
एतैः पापैर्न लिप्येत योनिमुद्रानिबन्धनात् ।।४३।।

यानि पापानि घोराणि तूपपापानि यानि च ।
तानि सर्वाणि नश्यन्ति योनिमुद्रानिबन्धनात् ।
तस्मादभ्यसनं कुर्याद्यदि मुक्तिं समिच्छति ।।४४।।

अथ वज्रोलीमुद्राकथनम् ।

आश्रित्य भूमिं करयोस्तलाभ्यामूर्ध्वं क्षिपेत्पादयुगं शिरः खे ।
शक्तिप्रबुद्धयै चिरजीवनाय वज्रोलिमुद्रां मुनयो वदन्ति ।।४५।।

अथ वज्रोलीमुद्रायाः फलकथनम् ।

योगश्रेष्ठो ह्ययं योगो योगिनां मुक्तिकारणम् ।
अयं हितप्रदो योगो योगिनां सिद्धिदायकः ।।४६।।

एतद्योगप्रसादेन बिन्दुसिद्धिर्भवेद् ध्रुवम् ।
सिद्धे बिन्दौ महायत्ने किं न सिध्यति भूतले ।।४७।।

भोगेन महता युक्तो यदि मुद्रां समाचरेत् ।
तथाऽपि सकला सिद्धिर्जायते तस्य निश्चितम् ॥४८॥

अथ शक्तिचालनीमुद्राकथनम् ।

मूलाधार आत्मशक्तिः कुण्डली परदेवता ।
शयिता भुजगाकारा सार्धत्रिवलयान्विता ॥४९॥

यावत्सा निद्रिता देहे तावज्जीवः पशुर्यथा ।
ज्ञानं न जायते तावत्कोटियोगं समभ्यसेत् ॥५०॥

उद्घाटयेत्कवाटं च तथा कुञ्चिकया हठात् ।
कुण्डलिन्याः प्रबोधेन ब्रह्मद्वारं प्रभेदयेत् ॥५१॥

नाभिं संवेष्ट्य वस्त्रेण न च नग्नो बहिःस्थितः ।
गोपनीयगृहे स्थित्वा शक्तिचालनमभ्यसेत् ॥५२॥

वितस्तिप्रमितं दीर्घं विस्तारे चतुरङ्गुलम् ।
मृदुलं धवलं सूक्ष्मं वेष्टनाम्बरलक्षणम् ।
एवमम्बरयुक्तं च कटिसूत्रेण योजयेत् ॥५३॥

संलिप्य भस्मना गात्रं सिद्धासनमथाचरेत् ।
नासाभ्यां प्राणमाकृष्याप्यपाने योजयेद् बलात् ॥५४॥

तावदाकुञ्चयेद् गुह्यमश्विनीमुद्रया शनैः ।
यावद्गच्छेत्सुषुम्णायां हठाद्वायुः प्रकाशयेत् ॥५५॥

तदा वायुप्रबन्धेन कुम्भिका च भुजङ्गिनी ।
बद्धश्वासस्ततो भूत्वा चोर्ध्वमार्गं प्रपद्यते ॥५६॥

विना शक्तिचालनेन योनिमुद्रा न सिध्यति ।
आदौ चालनमभ्यस्य योनिमुद्रां समभ्यसेत् ॥५७॥

इति ते कथितं चण्डकपाले शक्तिचालनम् ।
गोपनीयं प्रयत्नेन दिने दिने समभ्यसेत् ॥५८॥

अथ शक्तिचालनीमुद्रायाः फलकथनम् ।

मुद्रेयं परमा गोप्या जरामरणनाशिनी ।
तस्मादभ्यसनं कार्यं योगिभिः सिद्धिकाङ्क्षिभिः ॥५९॥

नित्यं योऽभ्यसते योगी सिद्धिस्तस्य करे स्थिता ।
तस्य विग्रहसिद्धिः स्याद्रोगाणां संक्षयो भवेत् ॥६०॥

अथ ताडागीमुद्राकथनम् ।

उदरं पश्चिमोत्तानं तडागाकृति कारयेत् ।
ताडागी सा परा मुद्रा जरामृत्युविनाशिनी ॥६१॥

अथ माण्डुकीमुद्राकथनम् ।

मुखं संमुद्रितं कृत्वा जिह्वामूलं प्रचालयेत् ।
शनैर्ग्रसेत्तदमृतं माण्डुकीं मुद्रिकां विदुः ।।६२।।

अथ माण्डुकीमुद्रायाः फलकथनम् ।

वलितं पलितं नैव जायते नित्ययौवनम् ।
न केशे जायते पाको यः कुर्यान्नित्यमाण्डुकीम् ।।६३।।

अथ शांभवीमुद्राकथनम् ।

नेत्रान्तरं समालोक्य चात्मारामं निरीक्षयेत् ।
सा भवेच्छांभवी मुद्रा सर्वतन्त्रेषु गोपिता ।।६४।।

अथ शांभवीमुद्रायाः फलकथनम् ।

वेदशास्त्रपुराणानि सामान्यगणिका इव ।
इयं तु शांभवी मुद्रा गुप्ता कुलवधूरिव ।।६५।।

स एव ह्यादिनाथश्च स च नारायणः स्वयम् ।
स च ब्रह्मा सृष्टिकारी यो मुद्रां वेत्ति शांभवीम् ।।६६।।

सत्यं सत्यं पुनः सत्यं सत्यमाह महेश्वरः ।
शांभवीं यो विजानीयात्स च ब्रह्म न चान्यथा ।।६७।।

अथ पञ्चधारणामुद्राकथनम् ।

कथिता शांभवी मुद्रा शृणुष्व पञ्चधारणाम् ।
धारणानि समासाद्य किं न सिध्यति भूतले ।।६८।।

अनेन नरदेहेन स्वर्गेषु गमनागमम् ।
मनोगतिर्भवेत्तस्य खेचरत्वं न चान्यथा ।।६९।।

अथ पार्थिवीधारणामुद्राकथनम् ।

यत्तत्त्वं हरितालदेशरचितं भौमं लकारान्वितं
वेदास्रं कमलासनेन सहितं कृत्वा हृदि स्थापितम् ।
प्राणं तत्र विलीय पञ्च घटिकाश्चित्तान्वितं धारयेदेषा
स्तम्भकरी सदा क्षितिजयं कुर्यादधोधारणा ।।७०।।

अथ पार्थिवीधारणामुद्रायाः फलकथनम् ।

पार्थिवीधारणामुद्रां यः करोति च नित्यशः ।
मृत्युंजयः स्वयं सोऽपि स सिद्धो विचरेद् भुवि ।।७१।।

अथ आम्भसीधारणामुद्राकथनम् ।

शङ्खेन्दुप्रतिमं च कुन्दधवलं तत्त्वं किलालं शुभं

तत्पीयूषवकारबीजसहितं युक्तं सदा विष्णुना ।
प्राणं तत्र विलीय पञ्च घटिकाश्चित्तान्वितं धारयेदेषा
दुःसहतापपापहरणी स्यादाम्भसी धारणा ॥७२॥

अथ आम्भसीमुद्रायाः फलकथनम् ।

आम्भसीं परमां मुद्रां यो जानाति स योगवित् ।
गभीरे च जले घोरे मरणं तस्य नो भवेत् ॥७३॥

इयं तु परमा मुद्रा गोपनीया प्रयत्नतः ।
प्रकाशात्सिद्धिहानिः स्यात्सत्यं वच्मि च तत्त्वतः ॥७४॥

अथ आग्नेयीधारणामुद्राकथनम् ।

यन्नाभिस्थितमिन्द्रगोपसदृशं बीजं त्रिकोणान्वितं
तत्त्वं वह्निमयं प्रदीप्तमरुणं रुद्रेण यत्सिद्धिदम् ।
प्राणं तत्र विलीय पञ्च घटिकाश्चित्तान्वितं धारयेदेषा
कालगभीरभीतिहरणी वैश्वानरी धारणा ॥७५॥

अथ आग्नेयीधारणामुद्रायाः फलकथनम् ।

प्रदीप्ते ज्वलिते वह्नावपि चेत्साधकः पतेत् ।
एतन्मुद्राप्रसादेन स जीवति न मृत्युभाक् ॥७६॥

अथ वायवीधारणामुद्राकथनम् ।

यद्भिन्नाञ्जनपुञ्जसंनिभमिदं धूम्रावभासं परं
तत्त्वं सत्त्वमयं यकारसहितं यत्रेश्वरो देवता ।
प्राणं तत्र विलीय पञ्च घटिकाश्चित्तान्वितं धारये-
देषा खे गमनं करोति यमिनां स्याद्वायवी धारणा ॥७७॥

अथ वायवीधारणामुद्रायाः फलकथनम् ।

इयं तु परमा मुद्रा जरामृत्युविनाशिनी ।
वायुना म्रियते नापि खे गतेश्च प्रदायिनी ॥७८॥

शठाय भक्तिहीनाय न देया यस्य कस्यचित् ।
दत्ते च सिद्धिहानिः स्यात्सत्यं वच्मि च चण्ड ते ॥७९॥

अथ आकाशीधारणामुद्राकथनम् ।

यत्सिन्धौ वरशुद्धवारिसदृशं व्योमाख्यमुद्भासते
तत्त्वं देवसदाशिवेन सहितं बीजं हकारान्वितम् ।
प्राणं तत्र विलीय पञ्च घटिकाश्चित्तान्वितं धारये-
देषा मोक्षकवाटभेदनकरी कुर्यान्नभोधारणाम् ॥८०॥

अथ आकाशीधारणामुद्रायाः फलकथनम् ।

आकाशीधारणां मुद्रां यो वेत्ति स च योगवित् ।
न मृत्युजरिते तस्य प्रलये नावसीदति ॥८१॥

अथ अश्विनीमुद्राकथनम् ।

आकुञ्चयेद् गुदद्वारं प्रकाशयेत्पुनः पुनः ।
सा भवेदश्विनीमुद्रा शक्तिप्रबोधकारिणी ॥८२॥

अश्विनीमुद्रायाः फलकथनम् ।

अश्विनी परमा मुद्रा गुह्यरोगविनाशिनी ।
बलपुष्टिकरी चैवाप्यकालमरणं हरेत् ॥८३॥

अथ पाशिनीमुद्राकथनम् ।

कण्ठपृष्ठे क्षिपेत्पादौ पाशवद् दृढबन्धनम् ।
सैव स्यात्पाशिनीमुद्रा शक्तिप्रबोधकारिणी ॥८४॥

अथ पाशिनीमुद्रायाः फलकथनम् ।

पाशिनी महती मुद्रा बलपुष्टिविधायिनी ।
साधनीया प्रयत्नेन साधकैः सिद्धिकाङ्क्षिभिः ॥८५॥

अथ काकीमुद्राकथनम् ।

काकचञ्चुवदास्येन पिबेद्वायुं शनैः शनैः ।
काकीमुद्रा भवेदेषा सर्वरोगविनाशिनी ॥८६॥

अथ काकीमुद्रायाः फलकथनम् ।

काकीमुद्रा परा मुद्रा सर्वतन्त्रेषु गोपिता ।
अस्याः प्रसादमात्रेण न रोगी काकवद् भवेत् ॥८७॥

अथ मातङ्गिनीमुद्राकथनम् ।

कण्ठदघ्ने जले स्थित्वा नासाभ्यां जलमाहरेत् ।
मुखान्निर्गमयेत्पश्चात्पुनर्वक्त्रेण चाहरेत् ॥८८॥
नासाभ्यां रेचयेत्पश्चात्कुर्यादेवं पुनः पुनः ।
मातङ्गिनी परा मुद्रा जरामृत्युविनाशिनी ॥८९॥

अथ मातङ्गिनीमुद्रायाः फलकथनम् ।

विरले निर्जने देशे स्थित्वा चैकाग्रमानसः ।
कुर्यान्मातङ्गिनीं मुद्रां मातङ्ग इव जायते ॥९०॥
यत्र यत्र स्थितो योगी सुखमत्यन्तमश्नुते ।
तस्मात्सर्वप्रयत्नेन साधयेन्मुद्रिकां पराम् ॥९१॥

अथ भुजङ्गिनीमुद्राकथनम् ।

वक्त्रं किंचित्सुप्रसार्य चानिलं गलया पिबेत् ।
सा भवेद् भुजगी मुद्रा जरामृत्युविनाशिनी ॥९२॥

अथ भुजङ्गिनीमुद्रायाः फलकथनम् ।

यावन्तश्चोदरे रोगा अजीर्णाद्या विशेषतः ।
तान्सर्वान्नाशयेवाशु यत्र मुद्रा भुजङ्गिनी ॥९३॥

इदं तु मुद्रापटलं कथितं चण्ड ते शुभम् ।
वल्लभं सर्वसिद्धानां जरामरणनाशनम् ॥९४॥

शठाय भक्तिहीनाय न देयं यस्य कस्यचित् ।
गोपनीयं प्रयत्नेन दुर्लभं मरुतामपि ॥९५॥

ऋजवे शान्तचित्ताय गुरुभक्तिपराय च ।
कुलीनाय प्रदातव्यं भोगमुक्तिप्रदायकम् ॥९६॥

मुद्राणां पटलं ह्येतत्सर्वव्याधिविनाशनम् ।
नित्यमभ्यासशीलस्य जाठराग्निविवर्धनम् ॥९७॥

न तस्य जायते मृत्युस्तथाऽस्य न जरादिकम् ।
नाग्निवारिभयं तस्य वायोरपि कुतो भयम् ॥९८॥

कासः श्वासः प्लीहा कुष्ठं श्लेष्मरोगाश्च विंशतिः ।
मुद्राणां साधनाच्चैव विनश्यन्ति न संशयः ॥९९॥

बहुना किमिहोक्तेन सारं वच्मि च चण्ड ते ।
नास्ति मुद्रासमं किंचित्सिद्धिदं क्षितिमण्डले ॥१००॥

इति श्रीघेरण्डसंहितायां घेरण्डचण्डसंवादे घटस्थ-
योगप्रकरणे मुद्राप्रयोगो नाम तृतीयोपदेशः ।

चतुर्थोपदेशः ।

घेरण्ड उवाच—

अथातः संप्रवक्ष्यामि प्रत्याहारकमुत्तमम् ।
यस्य विज्ञानमात्रेण कामादिरिपुनाशनम् ॥१॥

यतो यतो निश्चरति मनश्चञ्चलमस्थिरम् ।
ततस्ततो नियम्यैतदात्मन्येव वशं नयेत् ॥२॥

पुरस्कारं तिरस्कारं सुश्राव्यं वा भयानकम् ।
मनस्तस्मान्नियम्यैतदात्मन्येव वशं नयेत् ॥३॥

सुगन्धे वाऽपि दुर्गन्धे मनो घ्राणेषु जायते ।
तस्मात्प्रत्याहरेदेतदात्मन्येव वशं नयेत् ॥४॥

मधुराम्लकतिक्तादिरसं गतं यदा मनः ।
तस्मात्प्रत्याहरेदेतदात्मन्येव वशं नयेत् ॥५॥

इति श्रीघेरण्डसंहितायां घेरण्डचण्डसंवादे घटस्थ-
योगे प्रत्याहारप्रयोगो नाम चतुर्थोपदेशः ।

पञ्चमोपदेशः ।

घेरण्ड उवाच—

अथातः संप्रवक्ष्यामि प्राणायामस्य सद्विधिम् ।
यस्य साधनमात्रेण देवतुल्यो भवेन्नरः ॥१॥

आदौ स्थानं तथा कालं मिताहारं तथापरम् ।
नाडीशुद्धिं ततः पश्चात्प्राणायामं च साधयेत् ॥२॥

अथ स्थाननिर्णयः ।

दूरदेशे तथाऽरण्ये राजधान्यां जनान्तिके ।
योगारम्भं न कुर्वीत कृतश्चेत्सिद्धिहा भवेत् ॥३॥

अविश्वासं दूरदेशे अरण्ये रक्षिवर्जितम् ।
लोकारण्ये प्रकाशश्च तस्मात्त्रीणि विवर्जयेत् ॥४॥

सुदेशे धार्मिके राज्ये सुभिक्षे निरुपद्रवे ।
कृत्वा तत्रैकं कुटीरं प्राचीरैः परिवेष्टितम् ॥५॥

वापीकूपतडागं च प्राचीरमध्यवर्ति च ।
नात्युच्चं नातिनिम्नं च कुटीरं कीटवर्जितम् ॥६॥

सम्यग्गोमयलिप्तं च कुटीरं तत्र निर्मितम् ।
एवं स्थानेषु गुप्तेषु प्राणायामं समभ्यसेत् ॥७॥

अथ कालनिर्णयः ।

हेमन्ते शिशिरे ग्रीष्मे वर्षायां च ऋतौ तथा ।
योगारम्भं न कुर्वीत कृते योगो हि रोगदः ॥८॥

वसन्ते शरदि प्रोक्तं योगारम्भं समाचरेत् ।
तथा योगी भवेत्सिद्धो रोगान्मुक्तो भवेद् ध्रुवम् ।।९।।

चैत्रादिफाल्गुनान्ते च माघादिफाल्गुनान्तिके ।
द्वौ द्वौ मासावृतुभागावनुभावश्चतुश्चतुः ।।१०।।

वसन्तश्चैत्रवैशाखौ ज्येष्ठाषाढौ च ग्रीष्मकौ ।
वर्षा श्रावणभाद्राभ्यां शरदाश्विनकार्त्तिकौ ।
मार्गपौषौ च हेमन्तः शिशिरो माघफाल्गुनौ ।।११।।

अनुभावं प्रवक्ष्यामि ऋतूनां च यथोदितम् ।
माघादिमाधवान्तेषु वसन्तानुभवं विदुः ।।१२।।

चैत्रादि चाषाढान्तं च निदाघानुभवं विदुः ।
आषाढादि चाश्विनान्तं प्रावृषानुभवं विदुः ।।१३।।

भाद्रादि मार्गशीर्षान्तं शरदोऽनुभवं विदुः ।
कार्त्तिकान्माघमासान्तं हेमन्तानुभवं विदुः ।
मार्गादींश्चतुरो मासाञ्शिशिरानुभवं विदुः ।।१४।।

वसन्ते वाऽपि शरदि योगारम्भं समाचरेत् ।
तदा योगी भवेत्सिद्धो विनाऽऽयासेन कथ्यते ।।१५।।

अथ मिताहारः ।

मिताहारं विना यस्तु योगारम्भं तु कारयेत् ।
नानारोगो भवेत्तस्य किंचिद्योगो न सिध्यति ।।१६।।

शाल्यन्नं यवपिष्टं वा तथा गोधूमपिष्टकम् ।
मुद्गं माषचणकादि शुभ्रं च तुषवर्जितम् ।।१७।।

पटोलं पनसं मानं कक्कोलं च शुकाशकम् ।
द्राढिकां कर्कटीं रम्भां डुम्बरीं कण्टकण्टकम् ।।१८।।

आमरम्भां बालरम्भां रम्भावण्डं च मूलकम् ।
वार्ताकीं मूलकं चर्द्धि योगी भक्षणमाचरेत् ।।१९।।

बालशाकं कालशाकं तथा पटोलपत्रकम् ।
पञ्चशाकं प्रशंसीयाद्वास्तूकं हिमलोचिकाम् ।।२०।।

शुद्धं सुमधुरं स्निग्धमुदरार्धविवर्जितम् ।
भुज्यते सुरसं प्रीत्या मिताहारमिमं विदुः ।।२१।।

अन्नेन पूरयेदर्धं तोयेन तु तृतीयकम् ।
उदरस्य तुरीयांशं संरक्षेद्वायुचारणे ।।२२।।

कट्वम्लं लवणं तिक्तं भृष्टं च दधि तक्रकम् ।
शाकोत्कटं तथा मद्यं तालं च पनसं तथा ।।२३।।

कुलत्थं मसूरं पाण्डुं कूष्माण्डं शाकदण्डकम् ।
तुम्बीकोलकपित्थं च कण्टबिल्वं पलाशकम् ।।२४।।

कदम्बं जम्बीरं बिम्बं लकुचं लशुनं विषम् ।
कामरङ्गं पियालं च हिङ्गुशाल्मलिकेमुकम् ।।२५।।

योगारम्भे वर्जयेच्च पथिस्त्रीवह्निसेवनम् ।
नवनीतं घृतं क्षीरं शर्कराद्यैक्षवं गुडम् ।।२६।।

पक्वरम्भां नारिकेलं दाडिम्बमशिवासवम् ।
द्राक्षाङ्गुलवनीं धात्रीं रसमम्लविवर्जितम् ।।२७।।

एलाजातिलवङ्गं च पौरुषं जम्बु जाम्बवम् ।
हरीतकीं च खर्जूरं योगी भक्षणमाचरेत् ।।२८।।

लघुपाकं प्रियं स्निग्धं तथा धातुप्रपोषणम् ।
मनोभिलषितं योग्यं योगी भोजनमाचरेत् ।।२९।।

कठिनं दुरितं पूतिमुष्णं पर्युषितं तथा ।
अतिशीतं चातिचोष्णं भक्ष्यं योगी विवर्जयेत् ।।३०।।

प्रातःस्नानोपवासादि कायक्लेशविधिं तथा ।
एकाहारं निराहारं यामान्ते च न कारयेत् ।।३१।।

एवं विधिविधानेन प्राणायामं समाचरेत् ।
आरम्भे प्रथमे कुर्यात्क्षीराज्यं नित्यभोजनम् ।
मध्याह्ने चैव सायाह्ने भोजनद्वयमाचरेत् ।।३२।।

अथ नाडीशुद्धिः ।

कुशासने मृगाजिने व्याघ्राजिने च कम्बले ।
स्थलासने समासीनः प्राङ्मुखो वाऽप्युदङ्मुखः ।
नाडीशुद्धिं समासाद्य प्राणायामं समभ्यसेत् ।।३३।।

चण्डकापालिरुवाच ।

नाडीशुद्धिं कथं कुर्यान्नाडीशुद्धिस्तु कीदृशी ।
तत्सर्वं श्रोतुमिच्छामि तद्वदस्व दयानिधे ।।३४।।

घेरण्ड उवाच—

मलाकुलासु नाडीषु मारुतो नैव गच्छति ।
प्राणायामः कथं सिध्येत्तत्त्वज्ञानं कथं भवेत् ।
तस्मान्नाडीशुद्धिमादौ प्राणायामं ततोऽभ्यसेत् ।।३५।।

नाडीशुद्धिर्द्विधा प्रोक्ता समनुर्निर्मनुस्तथा ।
बीजेन समनुं कुर्यान्निर्मनुं धौतिकर्मणा ॥३६॥

धौतिकर्म पुरा प्रोक्तं षट्कर्मसाधने यथा ।
श्रृणुष्व समनुं चण्ड नाडीशुद्धिर्यथा भवेत् ॥३७॥

उपविश्यासने योगी पद्मासनं समाचरेत् ।
गुर्वादिन्यासनं कुर्याद्यथैव गुरुभाषितम् ।
नाडीशुद्धिं प्रकुर्वीत प्राणायामविशुद्धये ॥३८॥

वायुबीजं ततो ध्यात्वा धूम्रवर्णं सतेजसम् ।
चन्द्रेण पूरयेद्वायुं बीजं षोडशकैः सुधीः ॥३९॥

चतुःषष्ट्या मात्रया च कुम्भकेनैव धारयेत् ।
द्वात्रिंशन्मात्रया वायुं सूर्यनाड्या च रेचयेत् ॥४०॥

उत्थाप्याग्निं नाभिमूलाद् ध्यायेत्तेजोऽवनीयुतम् ।
वह्निबीजषोडशेन सूर्यनाड्या च पूरयेत् ॥४१॥

चतुःषष्ट्या मात्रया च कुम्भकेनैव धारयेत् ।
द्वात्रिंशन्मात्रया वायुं शशिनाड्या च रेचयेत् ॥४२॥

नासाग्रे शशधृग्बिम्बं ध्यात्वा ज्योत्स्नासमन्वितम् ।
ठं बीजं षोडशेनैव इडया पूरयेन्मरुत् ॥४३॥

चतुःषष्ट्या मात्रया च वं बीजेनैव धारयेत् ।
अमृतं प्लावितं ध्यात्वा नाडीधौतिं विभावयेत् ।
द्वात्रिंशेन लकारेण दृढं भाव्यं विरेचयेत् ॥४४॥

एवंविधां नाडीशुद्धिं कृत्वा नाडीं विशोधयेत् ।
दृढो भूत्वाऽऽसनं कृत्वा प्राणायामं समाचरेत् ॥४५॥

कुम्भकभेदाः ।

सहितः सूर्यभेदश्च उज्जायी शीतली तथा ।
भस्त्रिका भ्रामरी मूर्च्छा केवली चाष्ट कुम्भकाः ॥४६॥

सहितो द्विविधः प्रोक्तः सगर्भश्च निगर्भकः ।
सगर्भो बीजमुच्चार्य निगर्भो बीजवर्जितः ॥४७॥

प्राणायामं सगर्भं च प्रथमं कथयामि ते ।
सुखासने चोपविश्य प्राङ्मुखो वाऽप्युदङ्मुखः ।
रजोगुणं विधिं ध्यायेद्रक्तवर्णमवर्णकम् ॥४८॥

इडया पूरयेद्वायुं मात्रया षोडशैः सुधीः ।
पूरकान्ते कुम्भकाद्ये कर्तव्यस्तूड्डियानकः ॥४९॥

सत्त्वमयं हरिं ध्यात्वा उकारं कृष्णवर्णकम् ।
चतुःषष्टया च मात्रया कुम्भकेनैव धारयेत् ।।५०।।

तमोमयं शिवं ध्यात्वा मकारं शुक्लवर्णकम् ।
द्वात्रिंशन्मात्रया चैव रेचयेद्विधिना पुनः ।।५१।।

पुनः पिङ्गलयाऽऽपूर्य कुम्भकेनैव धारयेत् ।
इडया रेचयेत्पश्चात् तद्बीजेन क्रमेण तु ।।५२।।

अनुलोमविलोमेन वारं वारं च साधयेत् ।
पूरकान्ते कुम्भकान्तं धृतनासापुटद्वयम् ।
कनिष्ठानामिकाङ्गुष्ठैस्तर्जनीमध्यमे विना ।।५३।।

प्राणायामो निगर्भस्तु विना बीजेन जायते ।
वामजानूपरिन्यस्तवामपाणितलं भ्रमेत् ।
एकादिशतपर्यन्तं पूरकुम्भकरेचकम् ।।५४।।

उत्तमा विंशतिर्मात्रा षोडशी मात्रा मध्यमा ।
अधमा द्वादशी मात्रा प्राणायामास्त्रिधा स्मृताः ।।५५।।

अधमाज्जायते घर्मो मेरुकम्पश्च मध्यमात् ।
उत्तमाच्च भूमित्यागस्त्रिविधं सिद्धिलक्षणम् ।।५६।।

प्राणायामात्खेचरत्वं प्राणायामाद्रुजां हतिः ।
प्राणायामाच्छक्तिबोधः प्राणायामान्मनोन्मनी ।
आनन्दो जायते चित्ते प्राणायामी सुखी भवेत् ।।५७।।

अथ सूर्यभेदकुम्भकः ।

घेरण्ड उवाच—

कथितं सहितं कुम्भं सूर्यभेदनकं श्रृणु ।
पूरयेत्सूर्यनाड्या च यथाशक्ति बहिर्मरुत् ।।५८।।

धारयेद् बहुयत्नेन कुम्भकेन जलन्धरैः ।
यावत्स्वेदं नखकेशाभ्यां तावत्कुर्वन्तु कुम्भकम् ।।५९।।

प्राणोऽपानः समानश्चोदानव्यानौ तथैव च ।
नागः कूर्मश्च कृकरो देवदत्तो धनंजयः ।।६०।।

हृदि प्राणो वहेन्नित्यमपानो गुदमण्डले ।
समानो नाभिदेशे तु उदानः कण्ठमध्यगः ।।६१।।

व्यानो व्याप्य शरीरे तु प्रधानाः पञ्च वायवः ।
प्राणाद्याः पञ्च विख्याता नागाद्याः पञ्च वायवः ।।६२।।

तेषामपि च पञ्चानां स्थानानि च वदाम्यहम् ।
उद्गारे नाग आख्यातः कूर्मस्तून्मीलने स्मृतः ॥६३॥

कृकरः क्षुत्कृते ज्ञेयो देवदत्तो विजृम्भणे ।
न जहाति मृतं वाऽपि सर्वव्यापी धनंजयः ॥६४॥

नागो गृह्णाति चैतन्यं कूर्मश्चैव निमेषणम् ।
क्षुत्तृषं कृकरश्चैव चतुर्थेन तु जृम्भणम् ।
भवेद्धनंजयाच्छब्दः क्षणमात्रं न निःसरेत् ॥६५॥

सर्वे ते सूर्यसंभिन्ना नाभिमूलात्समुद्धरेत् ।
इडया रेचयेत्पश्चाद् धैर्येणाखण्डवेगतः ॥६६॥

पुनः सूर्येण चाकृष्य कुम्भयित्वा यथाविधि ।
रेचयित्वा साधयेत्तु क्रमेण च पुनः पुनः ॥६७॥

कुम्भकः सूर्यभेदस्तु जरामृत्युविनाशकः ।
बोधयेत्कुण्डलीं शक्तिं देहाग्निं च विवर्धयेत् ।
इति ते कथितं चण्ड सूर्यभेदनमुत्तमम् ॥६८॥

अथ उज्जायी कुम्भकः ।

नासाभ्यां वायुमाकृष्य मुखमध्ये च धारयेत् ।
हृद्गलाभ्यां समाकृष्य वायुं वक्त्रे च धारयेत् ॥६९॥

मुखं प्रक्षाल्य संवन्द्य कुर्याज्जालन्धरं ततः ।
आशक्ति कुम्भकं कृत्वा धारयेदविरोधतः ॥७०॥

उज्जायीकुम्भकं कृत्वा सर्वकार्याणि साधयेत् ।
न भवेत्कफरोगश्च क्रूरवायुरजीर्णकम् ॥७१॥

आमवातः क्षयः कासो ज्वरः प्लीहा न विद्यते ।
जरामृत्युविनाशाय चोज्जायीं साधयेन्नरः ॥७२॥

अथ शीतलीकुम्भकः ।

जिह्वया वायुमाकृष्य चोदरे पूरयेच्छनैः ।
क्षणं च कुम्भकं कृत्वा नासाभ्यां रेचयेत्पुनः ॥७३॥

सर्वदा साधयेद्योगी शीतलीकुम्भकं शुभम् ।
अजीर्णं कफपित्तं च नैव तस्य प्रजायते ॥७४॥

अथ भस्त्रिकाकुम्भकः ।

भस्त्रिका लोहकाराणां यथा क्रमेण संभ्रमेत् ।
तथा वायुं च नासाभ्यामुभाभ्यां चालयेच्छनैः ॥७५॥

एवं विंशतिवारं च कृत्वा कुर्याच्च कुम्भकम् ।
तदन्ते चालयेद्वायुं पूर्वोक्तं च यथाविधि ॥७६॥

त्रिवारं साधयेदेनं भस्त्रिकाकुम्भकं सुधीः ।
न च रोगो न च क्लेश आरोग्यं च दिने दिने ॥७७॥

अथ भ्रामरीकुम्भकः ।

अर्धरात्रे गते योगी जन्तूनां शब्दवर्जिते ।
कर्णौ पिधाय हस्ताभ्यां कुर्यात्पूरककुम्भकम् ॥७८॥

शृणुयाद्दक्षिणे कर्णे नादमन्तर्गतं शुभम् ।
प्रथमं झिल्लिकानादं वंशीनादं ततः परम् ॥७९॥

मेघझर्झरभ्रमरी घण्टा कांस्यं ततः परम् ।
तुरीभेरीमृदङ्गादिनिनादानकदुन्दुभिः ॥८०॥

एवं नानाविधो नादो जायते नित्यमभ्यसात् ।
अनाहतस्य शब्दस्य तस्य शब्दस्य यो ध्वनिः ॥८१॥

ध्वनेरन्तर्गतं ज्योतिर्ज्योतिरन्तर्गतं मनः ।
तन्मनो विलयं याति तद्विष्णोः परमं पदम् ।
एवं भ्रामरीसंसिद्धिः समाधिसिद्धिमाप्नुयात् ॥८२॥

अथ मूर्च्छाकुम्भकः ।

सुखेन कुम्भकं कृत्वा मनश्च भ्रुवोरन्तरम् ।
संत्यज्य विषयान्सर्वान्मनोमूर्च्छा सुखप्रदा ।
आत्मनि मनसो योगादानन्दो जायते ध्रुवम् ॥८३॥

अथ केवलीकुम्भकः ।

हंकारेण बहिर्याति सःकारेण विशेत्पुनः ।
षट्शतानि दिवारात्रौ सहस्राण्येकविंशतिः ।
अजपां नाम गायत्रीं जीवो जपति सर्वदा ॥८४॥

मूलाधारे यथा हंसस्तथा हि हृदि पङ्कजे ।
तथा नासापुटद्वन्द्वे त्रिभिर्हंससमागमः ॥८५॥

षण्णवत्यङ्गुलीमानं शरीरं कर्मरूपकम् ।
देहाद्बहिर्गतो वायुः स्वभावाद्द्वादशाङ्गुलिः ॥८६॥

गायने षोडशाङ्गुल्यो भोजने विंशतिस्तथा ।
चतुर्विंशाङ्गुलिः पन्थे निद्रायां त्रिंशदङ्गुलिः ।
मैथुने षट्त्रिंशदुक्तं व्यायामे च ततोऽधिकम् ॥८७॥

स्वभावेऽस्य गतेर्न्यूने परमायुः प्रवर्धते ।
आयुःक्षयोऽधिके प्रोक्तो मारुते चान्तराद्गते ।।८८।।

तस्मात्प्राणे स्थिते देहे मरणं नैव जायते ।
वायुना घटसंबन्धे भवेत्केवलकुम्भकम् ।।८९।।

यावज्जीवं जपेन्मन्त्रमजपासंख्यकेवलम् ।
अद्यावधि धृतं संख्याविभ्रमं केवलीकृते ।।९०।।

अत एव हि कर्तव्यः केवलीकुम्भको नरैः ।
केवली चाजपासंख्या द्विगुणा च मनोन्मनी ।।९१।।

नासाभ्यां वायुमाकृष्य केवलं कुम्भकं चरेत् ।
एकादिकचतुःषष्टिं धारयेत्प्रथमे दिने ।।९२।।

केवलीमष्टधा कुर्याद्यामे यामे दिने दिने ।
अथ वा पञ्चधा कुर्याद्यथा तत्कथयामि ते ।।९३।।

प्रातर्मध्याह्नसायाह्ने मध्येरात्रि चतुर्थके ।
त्रिसंध्यमथ वा कुर्यात्सममाने दिने दिने ।।९४।।

पञ्चवारं दिने वृद्धिर्वारैकं च दिने तथा ।
अजपापरिमाणं च यावत्सिद्धिः प्रजायते ।।९५।।

प्राणायामं केवली च तदा वदति योगवित् ।
केवलीकुम्भके सिद्धे किं न सिध्यति भूतले ।।९६।।

इति श्रीघेरण्डसंहितायां घेरण्डचण्डसंवादे घटस्थयोगप्रकरणे
प्राणायामप्रयोगो नाम पञ्चमोपदेशः ।

षष्ठोपदेशः

अथ ध्यानयोगः ।

घेरण्ड उवाच—

स्थूलं ज्योतिस्तथा सूक्ष्मं ध्यानस्य त्रिविधं विदुः ।
स्थूलं मूर्तिमयं प्रोक्तं ज्योतिस्तेजोमयं तथा ।
सूक्ष्मं बिन्दुमयं ब्रह्म कुण्डली परदेवता ।।१।।

अथ स्थूलध्यानम् ।

स्वकायहृदये ध्यायेत्सुधासागरमुत्तमम् ।
तन्मध्ये रत्नद्वीपं तु सुरत्नवालुकामयम् ।।२।।

चतुर्दिक्षु नीपतरुं बहुपुष्पसमन्वितम् ।
नीपोपवनसंकुलैर्वेष्टितं परिखा इव ॥३॥

मालतीमल्लिकाजातीकेसरैश्चम्पकैस्तथा ।
पारिजातैः स्थलपद्मैर्गन्धामोदितदिङ्मुखैः ॥४॥

तन्मध्ये संस्मरेद्योगी कल्पवृक्षं मनोहरम् ।
चतुःशाखाचतुर्वेदं नित्यपुष्पफलान्वितम् ॥५॥

भ्रमराः कोकिलास्तत्र गुञ्जन्ति निगदन्ति च ।
ध्यायेत्तत्र स्थिरो भूत्वा महामाणिक्यमण्डपम् ॥६॥

तन्मध्ये तु स्मरेद्योगी पर्यङ्कं सुमनोहरम् ।
तत्रेष्टदेवतां ध्यायेद्यद्ध्यानं गुरुभाषितम् ॥७॥

यस्य देवस्य यद्रूपं यथा भूषणवाहनम् ।
तद्रूपं ध्यायते नित्यं स्थूलध्यानमिदं विदुः ॥८॥

प्रकारान्तरम् ।

सहस्रारे महापद्मे कर्णिकायां विचिन्तयेत् ।
विलग्नसहितं पद्मं दलैर्द्वादशभिर्युतम् ॥९॥

शुक्लवर्णं महातेजो द्वादशैर्बीजभाषितम् ।
हसक्षमलवरयुं हसखफ्रें यथाक्रमम् ॥१०॥

तन्मध्ये कर्णिकायां तु अकथादिरेखात्रयम् ।
हळक्षकोणसंयुक्तं प्रणवं तत्र वर्तते ॥११॥

नादबिन्दुमयं पीठं ध्यायेत्तत्र मनोहरम् ।
तत्रोपरि हंसयुग्मं पादुका तत्र वर्तते ॥१२॥

ध्यायेत्तत्र गुरुं देवं द्विभुजं च त्रिलोचनम् ।
श्वेताम्बरधरं देवं शुक्लगन्धानुलेपनम् ॥१३॥

शुक्लपुष्पमयं माल्यं रक्तशक्तिसमन्वितम् ।
एवंविधगुरुध्यानात्स्थूलध्यानं प्रसिध्यति ॥१४॥

अथ ज्योतिर्ध्यानम् ।

घेरण्ड उवाच—

स्थूलध्यानं तु कथितं तेजोध्यानं शृणुष्व मे ।
यद्ध्यानेन योगसिद्धिरात्मप्रत्यक्षमेव च ॥१५॥

मूलाधारे कुण्डलिनी भुजगाकाररूपिणी ।
तत्र तिष्ठति जीवात्मा प्रदीपकलिकाकृतिः ।
ध्यायेत्तेजोमयं ब्रह्म तेजोध्यानं परात्परम् ॥१६॥

प्रकारान्तरम् ।

भ्रुवोर्मध्ये मनऊर्ध्वे यत्तेजः प्रणवात्मकम् ।
ध्यायेज्ज्वालावलीयुक्तं तेजोध्यानं तदेव हि ॥१७॥

अथ सूक्ष्मध्यानम् ।

घेरण्ड उवाच—

तेजोध्यानं श्रुतं चण्ड सूक्ष्मध्यानं श्रृणुष्व मे ।
बहुभाग्यवशाद्यस्य कुण्डली जाग्रती भवेत् ॥१८॥
आत्मना सह योगेन नेत्ररन्ध्राद्विनिर्गता ।
विहरेद्राजमार्गे च चञ्चलत्वान्न दृश्यते ॥१९॥
शांभवीमुद्रया योगी ध्यानयोगेन सिध्यति ।
सूक्ष्मध्यानमिदं गोप्यं देवानामपि दुर्लभम् ॥२०॥
स्थूलध्यानाच्छतगुणं तेजोध्यानं प्रचक्षते ।
तेजोध्यानाल्लक्षगुणं सूक्ष्मध्यानं परात्परम् ॥२१॥
इति ते कथितं चण्ड ध्यानयोगं सुदुर्लभम् ।
आत्मा साक्षाद्भवेद्यस्मात्तस्माद्ध्यानं विशिष्यते ॥२२॥

इति श्रीघेरण्डसंहितायां घेरण्डचण्डसंवादे घटस्थयोगे
सप्तमसाधने ध्यानयोगो नाम षष्ठोपदेशः ।

सप्तमोपदेशः ।

अथ समाधियोगः ।

घेरण्ड उवाच—

समाधिश्च परो योगो बहुभाग्येन लभ्यते ।
गुरोः कृपाप्रसादेन प्राप्यते गुरुभक्तितः ॥१॥
विद्याप्रतीतिः स्वगुरुप्रतीतिरात्मप्रतीतिर्मनसः प्रबोधः ।
दिने दिने यस्य भवेत्स योगी सुशोभनाभ्यासमुपैति सद्यः ॥२॥
घटाद्भिन्नं मनः कृत्वा चैक्यं कुर्यात्परात्मनि ।
समाधिं तं विजानीयान्मुक्तसंज्ञो दशादिभिः ॥३॥
अहं ब्रह्म न चान्योऽस्मि ब्रह्मैवाहं न शोकभाक् ।
सच्चिदानन्दरूपोऽहं नित्यमुक्तः स्वभाववान् ॥४॥

शांभव्या चैव खेचर्या भ्रामर्या योनिमुद्रया ।
ध्यानं नादं रसानन्दं लयसिद्धिश्चतुर्विधा ॥५॥

पञ्चधा भक्तियोगेन मनोमूर्च्छा च षड्विधा ।
षड्विधोऽयं राजयोगः प्रत्येकमवधारयेत् ॥६॥

अथ ध्यानयोगसमाधिः ।

शांभवीं मुद्रिकां कृत्वा आत्मप्रत्यक्षमानयेत् ।
बिन्दुं ब्रह्ममयं दृष्ट्वा मनस्तत्र नियोजयेत् ॥७॥

खमध्ये कुरु चात्मानमात्ममध्ये च खं कुरु ।
आत्मानं खमयं दृष्ट्वा न किंचदपि बुध्यते ।
सदाऽऽनन्दमयो भूत्वा समाधिस्थो भवेन्नरः ॥८॥

अथ नादयोगसमाधिः ।

खेचरीमुद्रासाधनाद् रसनोर्ध्वगता यदा ।
तदा समाधिसिद्धिः स्याद्धित्वा साधारणक्रियाम् ॥९॥

अथ रसनानन्दयोगसमाधिः ।

अनिलं मन्दवेगेन भ्रामरीकुम्भकं चरेत् ।
मन्दं मन्दं रेचयेद्वायुं भृङ्गनादं ततो भवेत् ॥१०॥

अन्तःस्थं भ्रमरीनादं श्रुत्वा तत्र मनो नयेत् ।
समाधिर्जायते तत्र चानन्दः सोऽहमित्यतः ॥११॥

अथ लयसिद्धियोगसमाधिः ।

योनिमुद्रां समासाद्य स्वयं शक्तिमयो भवेत् ।
सुश्रृङ्गाररसेनैव विहरेत्परमात्मनि ॥१२॥

आनन्दमयः संभूत्वा ऐक्यं ब्रह्मणि संभवेत् ।
अहं ब्रह्मेति चाद्वैतसमाधिस्तेन जायते ॥१३॥

अथ भक्तियोगसमाधिः ।

स्वकीयहृदये ध्यायेदिष्टदेवस्वरूपकम् ।
चिन्तयेद्भक्तियोगेन परमाह्लादपूर्वकम् ॥१४॥

आनन्दाश्रुपुलकेन दशाभावः प्रजायते ।
समाधिः संभवेत्तेन संभवेच्च मनोन्मनी ॥१५॥

अथ राजयोगसमाधिः ।

मनोमूर्च्छां समासाद्य मन आत्मनि योजयेत् ।
परात्मनः समायोगात्समाधिं समवाप्नुयात् ॥१६॥

अथ समाधियोगमाहात्म्यम् ।

इति ते कथितश्चण्ड समाधिर्मुक्तिलक्षणम् ।
राजयोगसमाधिः स्यादेकात्मन्येव साधनम् ।
उन्मनी सहजावस्था सर्वे चैकात्मवाचकाः ।।१७।।

जले विष्णुः स्थले विष्णुर्विष्णुः पर्वतमस्तके ।
ज्वालामालाकुले विष्णुः सर्वं विष्णुमयं जगत् ।।१८।।

भूचराः खेचराश्चामी यावन्तो जीवजन्तवः ।
वृक्षगुल्मलतावल्लीतृणाद्या वारि पर्वताः ।
सर्वं ब्रह्म विजानीयात्सर्वं पश्यति चात्मनि ।।१९।।

आत्मा घटस्थचैतन्यमद्वैतं शाश्वतं परम् ।
घटाद्विभिन्नतो ज्ञात्वा वीतरागं विवासनम् ।।२०।।

एवं मिथः समाधिः स्यात्सर्वसंकल्पवर्जितः ।
स्वदेहे पुत्रदारादिबान्धवेषु धनादिषु ।
सर्वेषु निर्ममो भूत्वा समाधिं समवाप्नुयात् ।।२१।।

तत्त्वं लयामृतं गोप्यं शिवोक्तं विविधानि च ।
तेषां संक्षेपमादाय कथितं मुक्तिलक्षणम् ।।२२।।

इति ते कथितश्चण्ड समाधिर्दुर्लभः परः ।
यं ज्ञात्वा न पुनर्जन्म जायते भूमिमण्डले ।।२३।।

इति श्रीघेरण्डसंहितायां घेरण्डचण्डसंवादे घटस्थयोगसाधने योगस्य
सप्तसारे समाधियोगो नाम सप्तमोपदेशः समाप्तः ।

ERRATA

Page	Read	For
64	Adopting	Adcpting
104	dioica	dioeca
140	Tantric	Tāntric
162	ऊर्ध्वा	उर्ध्वा
172	यानि	थानि
175	कुर्यान्नभोधारणाम्	कुयार्न्नभोधारणाम्
179	चर्द्धि	चर्द्वि

Yoni Linga
Mudra

Sambhavi
mudra
(eyes)